Recent Advances in Audiological and Vestibular Research

Edited by Stavros Hatzopoulos and Andrea Ciorba

Published in London, United Kingdom

Recent Advances in Audiological and Vestibular Research
http://dx.doi.org/10.5772/intechopen.102239
Edited by Stavros Hatzopoulos and Andrea Ciorba

Contributors
Raheel Ahmed, Rumana Ahmed, Sergio Masetto, Paolo Spaiardi, Stuart J. Johnson, Başak Mutlu, Maoli Duan, Wen Xie, Moslem Shaabani, Madalina Georgescu, Magdalena B. Skarżyńska

First published in London, United Kingdom, 2022 by IntechOpen
IntechOpen is the global imprint of INTECHOPEN LIMITED, registered in England and Wales, registration number: 11086078, 5 Princes Gate Court, London, SW7 2QJ, United Kingdom

British Library Cataloguing-in-Publication Data
A catalogue record for this book is available from the British Library

Additional hard and PDF copies can be obtained from orders@intechopen.com

Recent Advances in Audiological and Vestibular Research
Edited by Stavros Hatzopoulos and Andrea Ciorba
p. cm.
Print ISBN 978-1-80356-374-9
Online ISBN 978-1-80356-375-6
eBook (PDF) ISBN 978-1-80356-376-3

Meet the editors

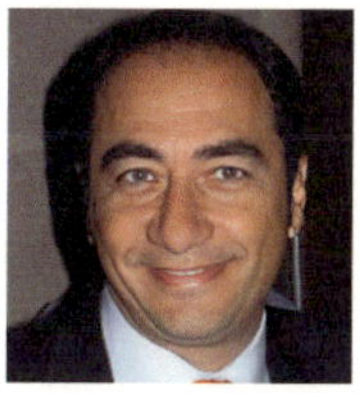

Dr. Stavros Hatzopoulos has been a faculty member of the Audiology & ENT Clinic, at the University of Ferrara, Italy, since 1994. His background is in biomedical, engineering, audiological engineering, and hearing science (BSc degree from the University of Southern California, MSc from Texas A&M, Ph.D. from Worcester Polytechnic Institute in Massachusetts). He received his habilitation as an associate professor in 2014. He is the author of more than 225 book chapters, peer review papers, and congress presentations. He has participated in numerous European Concerted Action projects in the areas of otoacoustic emissions, genetics, and nanotechnologies. He currently serves as the editor of the Portal on Otoacoustic Emissions (www.otoemissions.org), as the Audiology section editor for the journal of Hearing Science and as the Managing editor for the Journal of Hearing, Balance & Communication.

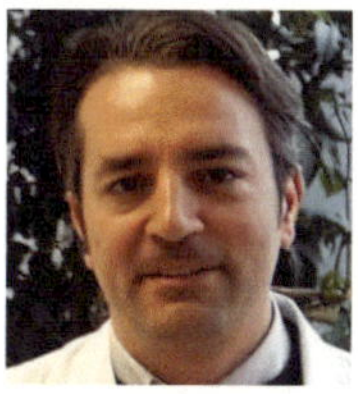

Dr. Andrea Ciorba, MD, has been a member of the Audiology & ENT Clinic, at the University of Ferrara, Italy, since 2004. He is the author of about 190 peer-reviewed papers and book chapters, and he is a member of the editorial boards of several peer-reviewed journals. His clinical field of interest is audiology and vestibology, and he is also involved in research activities in the field of otoacoustic emissions and inner ear electrophysiology. After earning his degree in Medicine in 1999 and a Diploma in Otolaryngology and Head and Neck Surgery in October 2003, he obtained a Ph.D. in Audiology in March 2008. Since November 2020, he is an Associate Professor of Audiology at the Audiology & ENT Clinic, at the University of Ferrara, Italy.

Contents

Preface

This book provides information on the latest research and findings on the vestibular system, the apparatus of the inner ear involved in the maintenance of balance perception. The correct evaluation and identification of vestibular diseases are important to achieving correct rehabilitation and restoration of the balance function.

Vestibular research, although quite important, is not the main player in audiological research, and very often important vestibular topics and arguments do not receive the necessary attention from the scientific community. For example, after the two-year COVID-19 dominion on virally transmitted diseases, the PRISMA review data we had collected in Italy and Europe referred to a symptomatology related more to the inner than the middle ear, with a clear preference for sudden hearing losses (SNHL) than vertigo and tinnitus [1].

After the recent COVID-19 mass vaccinations, a series of adverse side effects were widely reported, including audio-vestibular symptoms. Our team followed these reports in Italy and the United Kingdom and published a paper [2] showing that vestibular symptoms were the most reported side effects along with the sensation of tinnitus. We were advised by the Italian and UK authorities that we could not suggest a clear correlation between the reported audio-vestibular symptoms and the applied vaccination policies. This argument is still open though because the number of reports in the Italian Association of Pharmacology database (AIFA) is considered significant, that is, there is a greater volume of complaints related to COVID vaccinations compared to the side effects reported from the use of traditional vaccines and vaccination policies. However, the reader should acknowledge that the high number of audio-vestibular adverse effects could be the result of the extremely large volume of vaccines applied for the first time on such a broad human scale.

This book was made possible through the substantial contribution of numerous authors. It is designed for students in otolaryngology, audiology, speech pathology, hearing science, and neurosciences, among others.

The material of this volume is divided into two sections: “Vestibular Pathophysiological Features” and “Updates on Diagnosis and Therapy.”

Section 1 discusses several aspects of the vestibular system, particularly the pathophysiology of the vestibular pathways. Chapters in this part discuss the latest advances in hearing loss and vestibular disorders in children, tinnitus, and stem cell and gene therapies.

- Chapter 1: “Advances in Hearing Loss and Vestibular Disorders in Children”

- Chapter 2: “Evidence of a Neuroinflammatory Model of Tinnitus”

- Chapter 3: "Signal Transmission by Auditory and Vestibular Hair Cells"

Section 2 provides updates on several innovative approaches for the modern evaluation and rehabilitation of vestibular disorders. Chapters in this part discuss vestibular therapy, rehabilitation, testing, and the possible association of audio-vestibular side effects and COVID-19 treatments.

- Chapter 4: "Vestibular Therapy"
- Chapter 5: "Vestibular Rehabilitation: Conventional and Virtual Reality-Based Methods"
- Chapter 6: "Hearing and Vestibular Testing in Meniere's Disease"
- Chapter 7: "Audio-Vestibular Side Effects of Drugs and Vaccines in Treatment of COVID-19"

We would like to thank all the authors for their excellent contributions. We are also grateful to the staff at IntechOpen for their continuous and generous assistance during the preparation of this book.

Stavros Hatzopoulos, Ph.D.
Audiology & ENT Clinic,
University of Ferrara,
Ferrara, Italy

Andrea Ciorba, MD, Ph.D.
Audiology & ENT Clinic,
University of Ferrara,
Ferrara, Italy

References

[1] Fancello V, Hatzopoulos S, Corazzi V, Bianchini C, Skarżyńska MB, Pelucchi S, Skarżyński PH, Ciorba A. Sars-C0r-2 (COVID-19) and Audio-Vestibular disorders. International Journal of Immunopathology and Pharmacology. Jan-Dec 2021;**34**. DOI: 10.1177/2058738420941754

[2] Ciorba A, Bianchini C, Caranti A, Skarżyński PH, Pelucchi S, Hatzopoulos S. Audiological adverse effects after Covid-19 vaccination. A Preliminary Study. Ear Nose & Throat. Sept 2021. DOI : 10.1177/01455613211048975

Section 1

Vestibular Pathophysiological Features

Chapter 1

Advances in Hearing Loss and Vestibular Disorders in Children

Wen Xie and Maoli Duan

Abstract

Pediatric hearing loss is a common sensory deficit, affecting nearly 9% of children worldwide. Compared with pediatric hearing loss, vestibular disorders are still not known among the child population. However, vestibular disorders are more and more generally known with time when the measurement of vestibular function is developing. Genetic causes and virus infection are the main causes of pediatric hearing loss, and vestibular migraine is the most common etiological disease of childhood vertigo. This narrative review of the literature discusses the brief etiopathology, the clinical manifestations of hearing loss and vestibular disorders in children, as well as available test protocols to diagnose childhood hearing loss and vestibular dysfunction.

Keywords: hearing loss, vestibular disorders, child, auditory tests, vestibular tests

1. Introduction

Hearing loss is a common sensory deficit in children, nearly 9% of hearing loss occurs in children worldwide [1], and 1–3 out of 1000 deliveries suffer from permanent hearing loss worldwide [2, 3]. Hearing loss has detriment impact on children's quality of life. It may affect children's speech and language development, as well as their learning ability and school performance consequently. Moreover, their cognitive, social, and psychosocial development may be negatively affected [4]. Over the past 30 years, the understanding of the etiology of pediatric hearing loss experienced a steady growth, and the diagnosis and treatment technology for pediatric hearing loss witness a huge development. However, infants with hearing impairment may behavior normally. They soon present hearing difficulty or speech and language delay with time. Therefore, identifying the hearing using newborns universal hearing screening is essential. On the other hand, some children may pass the hearing screening but suffer from delayed-onset hearing loss. Thus, continuous surveillance of their hearing and the speech-language development are essential.

The relationship between auditory and vestibular function is close, children with hearing loss may combined with vertigo or imbalance, due to the anatomy adjacency between the auditory organs and vestibular end-organs. The estimated prevalence of vestibular dysfunction ranges between 0.4 and 8% [5, 6]. Compared with pediatric hearing loss, published medical literature on pediatric vestibular disorders is scant. Vestibular disorders can have significant impacts on children's quality of life. It may lead to delayed motor skills, attention deficit disorder, learning problems, developmental delay, intellectual disability and emotional disorders [7]. With the increasing awareness of the harm of vestibular disorders in children, more and more studies focus on this field recently. Currently, there are several challenges in the study of childhood vestibular disorders. Firstly, the inability of children to explain the characteristics of the vertigo symptoms make the diagnosis of vestibular disease difficult, especially in very young children. In addition, due to poor cooperation, the vestibular tests are not uniformly reliable in the younger pediatric patients.

We will focus causes of pediatric hearing loss and vestibular disorders, and introduce the advance in the technology of the common auditory, molecular test and vestibular evaluation protocols in children with hearing loss and/or vestibular disorders.

2. Causes of pediatric hearing loss

Pediatric hearing loss is either congenital or acquired. The causes of congenital hearing loss are various, including congenital cytomegalovirus infection, genetic, anatomical abnormalities of the ears. The causes of postnatal acquired hearing loss can be attributed to genetic, trauma, infection, or ototoxic medications [8]. Risk indicators of childhood later-one onset hearing loss include caregivers' concern, family history, findings associated with sensorineural hearing loss (SNHL), hyperbilirubinemia, neurodegenerative disorders and otitis media with effusion [9, 10].

3. Congenital hearing loss

3.1 Virus infection

It is estimated that the 5–20% of congenital hearing loss is caused by congenital cytomegalovirus (CMV) infection [8], which occurs in 0.4–0.64% of all newborns [11, 12]. Clinical spectrum of congenital CMV infection varies widely, 85–90% of infected infants are complete absence of signs of infection (asymptomatic infection). Thus, it is best for all asymptomatic newborns with suspicion of CMV infection undergo either universal or targeted screening of CMV. However, due to the concern of cost, newborn screening for CMV is not widely applied worldwide.

Up to 10–15% children with CMV infection exhibit apparent infection manifestation (symptomatic disease), among them, some infants may present with potentially life-threatening disseminated disease [11, 13]. The common presentation of the CMV infection in symptomatic children are petechiae, jaundice, hepatomegaly, splenomegaly, microcephaly, and other neurologic signs. Among infants who develop CMV-related SNHL, hearing loss may occur at birth or later [14]. Moreover, about 50% of children with SNHL following CMV will continue to have further hearing loss deterioration or progression [15, 16]. Therefore, it is important for all infants with congenital CMV infection, whether they having hearing loss or not, receive serial audiological monitoring throughout the first year of life to allow for early detection of possible SNHL. Other known congenital infections that may cause neonatal hearing loss are TORCH microorganisms (toxoplasmosis, other organisms, rubella, CMV, herpes) [9].

3.2 Genetic causes

The majority of congenital hearing loss, up to 60% of cases, is due to a genetic etiology [17]. The genetic phenotypes of SNHL can be defined as syndromic or non-syndromic. 70% of newborns Hearing loss is non-syndromic. Up to now, 124 genes are found to be associated with non-syndromic hearing loss [18]. Most of the patients with non-syndromic SNHL have the disease-causing variant in the gene GJB2, which encodes the protein connexin 26 [19]. Hearing loss due to GJB2 deficiency was first reported in 1997. Now, various gene variances are reported to be related to the onset of hearing loss. 80% of non-syndromic genetic hearing loss is caused by autosomal-recessive (AR) inheritance, predominantly occurs prelingually and frequently results in severe hearing loss [20]. On the other hand, autosomal-dominant (AD) inheritance accounts for most of the other 20% of non-syndromic genetic hearing loss and more often result in variable level of progressive hearing loss and occurs between 10 and 40 years old [21].

The remaining 30% of congenital hearing loss present with syndromic form and is associated with structural or functional anomalies of other organs and systems [22]. Patients with mitochondrial inheritance predominately have variable severity of progressive SNHL, with onset aged between 5 and 50 years [23]. X-linked and mitochondrial inheritance accounts for only 1–2% of non-syndromic hearing loss [20].

More than 40 known genes are related to syndromic hearing loss [18]. Syndromic hearing loss may also be transmitted as an AR, AD, X-linked, or matrilineal trait [18]. Pendred, Usher, and Alport syndromes are the most common syndromic hearing loss among children. Pendred syndrome, cause by recessive variants in the SLC26A4 gene, is characterized by thyroid dysfunction, goiter, enlarged vestibular aqueduct, and incomplete partition type II cochlear abnormality (Mondini). Usher syndrome is associated with at least 9 genes and present with hearing loss, vestibular dysfunction, and vision loss. Alport syndromeisan X-linked (80%) or recessive disorder (depending on the gene) exhibit kidney failure, ocular abnormalities (anterior lenticonus, retinopathy), and progressive SNHL. It is noteworthy for patients with suspected syndromic hearing loss, it is even more important to identify the genetic cause, as many of the comorbidities can be more severe [24]. In brief, if a child has a three-generational family history suggestive of AD inheritance, a genetic cause is essentially established [25]. In addition, a comprehensive and thorough medical history collection and physical examination are needed for all hearing loss newborns to identify the insidious and harmful comorbidities.

4. Acquired hearing loss

Genetic causes, trauma, infection, or ototoxic medications are the main causes of acquired hearing loss. Genetic hearing loss, may occur later in childhood. For children with delayed hearing loss, genetic causes should always be considered, especially if other causes are excluded.

Environment causes leading acquired hearing loss include trauma, infection, exposure to ototoxic medications, chemotherapy and radiation therapy and noise. Of all of these, environmental noise is the most common cause of hearing loss [25].

Infectious causes of hearing loss can occur both before and after birth. As we mentioned previously, CMV is a substantial cause of delayed hearing loss in children. Other infectious causes of SNHL include measles, mumps, varicella zoster, Lyme disease, bacterial meningitis, and otitis media. Several groups of drugs are the well-recognized causes of SNHL, including aminoglycoside antibiotics, systemic chemotherapy (especially cisplatin), macrolides, and loop Kenna diuretics [26].

Furthermore, it is worth mentioning that otitis media is a common cause of pediatric hearing loss. OME is a middle ear disease that affects 90% of children at least once before they reach school age [27]. Although OME is very common in children, permanent SNHL caused by OME is rare. Persistent middle ear effusion is frequently found in children after the resolution of acute inflammation in acute otitis media.

5. The test batteries for diagnosing pediatric hearing loss

5.1 Auditory tests

For all newborn infants, neonatal hearing screening is essential. In 2000 and 2007, The Joint Committee on Infant Hearing (JCIH) recommended universal newborn hearing screening (UNHS) for newborn infants, in order to early detection of and intervention for infants with hearing loss [9]. Now, UNHS is applied in most developed countries, and these countries have formulated guideline for newborn hearing screening. Diverse screening protocols may be adopted in different countries. All these protocols are based on the 1-3-6 benchmark (screening completed by 1 month, audiological diagnosis by 3 month, enrolment in early intervention by 6 month) set in the earlier editions of the JCIH recommendations. Although UNHS is applied widely, many countries still do not have UNHS included in their health agenda, partly due to its high cost or doubt of its value [28].

The most common available newborns hearing screening tests to date include otoacoustic emissions (OAE), that is further classified as transient-evoked otoacoustic emissions (TEOAE) or distortion product otoacoustic emissions (DPOAE), and automated auditory brainstem response (aABR).

Children who fail the hearing screen should undergo further auditory test. Frequency-specific audiometry and tympanometry are considered to be the basic hearing tests for pediatric patients. However, additional behavioral and objective measures are essential to evaluate the hearing, and cross-check of subjective and objective hearing tests is needed to ensure an accurate and timely diagnosis. This is particularly important in the pediatric population [29].

Once the children are diagnosed with hearing loss, they will refer to the otorhinolaryngology specialists and audiologists to identify the etiology and receive treatment.

One problem must be considered is that a passed UNHS does not exclude a future delayed hearing loss onset, particularly in children with risk factors [30]. Therefore, it is necessary to continuously monitor their hearing and behavior, and children who have delayed speech and language development should be subjected to new hearing tests.

5.2 Molecular test

Any infant or child with bilateral congenital hearing loss of unknown etiology requires a genetics consultation and undergo genetic tests. For children with a suspicion of AR NSHL, genetic testing for GJB2 by Sanger sequencing is recommended [31]. In addition, serologic testing in both mother and infant is advised upon the suspicion of a congenital infection of CMV, toxoplasmosis, rubella, herpes simplex and syphilis [32].

At first, the only available genetic testing for hearing loss was single-gene testing. Now, comprehensive genetic testing (CGT) is becoming the new standard, this technology improves the genetic diagnostic yield by applying massively parallel sequencing or next generation sequencing (NGS), which make the cost of sequencing decrease and avoid multiple tests [33, 34].

Whole Genome Sequencing (WGS) is an emerging tool with the potential to generate an incomparable variety and quantities of genetic information. Although WES has shown to be a potential tool for DNA diagnostics of hearing loss, its sensitivity is lower than the targeted resequencing methods [35]. Moreover, the cost of WGS is relatively high, which limits its clinical application. Now, as the cost WGS is decreased, it is expected to be the standard diagnostic tool in clinical practice within 5 years [36].

Currently, the testing of congenital CMV infection in most highly resourced countries is based on clinical suspicion alone. This means a large proportion of CMV infections are underdiagnosed. Universal or targeted screening of CMV contributes to identify CMV infection, however, due to the cost concern, only infants with suspicious CMV undergo screening in most countries.

When pediatric patients are diagnosed with hearing loss. Standard examinations include history taking, physical examination and other examination can be selected according to their corresponding clinical manifestations. For example, computed tomography imaging or magnetic resonance imaging of temporal bone can be taken into consideration to exclude structural inner ear or neurological anomalies. Upon the suspicion of other syndromic hearing loss, different additional corresponding examinations can be performed according to the diagnosis, such as an electrocardiogram for Lange-Nielsen syndrome or a urine analysis and renal ultrasound for branchio-oto-renal syndrome [37, 38]. Ophthalmic examination is also necessary since the prevalence of ophthalmic problems in children with hearing loss is 40 to 60% [39]. In addition, vestibular evaluation should be performed in case of a negative result for both genetic and serologic tests in the sporadic cases or patients with a suspicion of AR SNHL [40].

6. Disease spectrum of pediatric vestibular disorders

The reported prevalence and etiologies of vestibular disorders are various depending on the medical institution which children are referred to, the referral criteria, the age range when they tested and the type of the vestibular testing they undergo [41]. According to a systematic review conducted by Brodsky et al., the top 4 diseases resulting in childhood vertigo were vestibular migraine (VM) (23.8%), benign paroxysmal vertigo of childhood (BPVC) (13.7%), idiopathic (11.7%), and labyrinthitis/vestibular neuronitis (8.47%). Less common etiological diseases included Meniere disease and central nervous system tumors [42]. Another recent clinical study also showed that the most common etiological diseases are VM and BPVC, followed by vestibular neuritis [43]. However, Gedik-Soyuyuce et al. pointed out that benign paroxysmal positional vertigo (BPPV) was the most common cause (49%), followed by VM (41%), BPVC (4.5%), vestibular neuritis (4.5%) and psychogenic vertigo (4.5%) [44].

Božanić Urbančič et al. investigated 257 vertigo/dizziness children and reported that central diseases accounted for 19.1%, peripheral vestibular diseases 12.4%, hemodynamic diseases 10.9%, and psychological diseases 5.8%. None of the symptoms were attributed to visual problems. 40.8% children with central vertigo had BPVC and 8.2% had migrainous vertigo. The etiology could not be identified among

112 children (43.6%) [45]. Moreover, they found the most common etiological central diseases is BPVC, other diseases such as epileptic, infectious, neoplastic, vascular, postoperative vertigo, vertigo due to hydrocephalus, degenerative/hereditary vertigo can also lead to vestibular symptoms.

To sum up, VM and BPVC are reported to be the most common causes of vertigo in children. VM is a subtype of migraine and is also common among adults. The speculated cause of migraine is the dysfunction of thalamocortical networks, which is vulnerable to trigger factors, including stressful life events, visual stimuli, hormonal changes, hypoglycaemia, or sleep deprivation [46]. In the developing brain, migraine may have a different phenotype than it does in the adult brain. For example, the duration of migraine attacks can be shorter in children, and the head pain is most often bilateral instead of unilateral. In some cases, children with migraine may not even exhibit headache [47]. BPVC is the early stage of VM, the reported prevalence of BPVC is variable, ranging from 6–20% [48]. Recently, the Committee for the Classification of Vestibular Disorders of the Bárány Society put forward the diagnostic criteria for Vestibular Migraine of Childhood [49]. The clinical presentation of BPVC is episodes of vertigo that typically last for minutes at a time and resolve spontaneously without any postictal symptoms.

Other reported common causes of pediatric vertigo include trauma, ocular disorders (such as vergence insufficiency, ametropia, anisometropia), congenital malformations and syndromes (Large vestibular aqueduct syndrome and Cogan syndrome), superior semicircular canal dehiscence, chronic otitis media and cholesteatoma, psychiatric disorders, central nervous system disorders (epilepsy, multiple sclerosis and episodic ataxia) and posterior fossa lesions (Vestibular schwannoma and Meningiomas) [50].

Persistent postural-perceptual dizziness (PPPD) is not as common in childhood as in adult age, Wang et al. Retrospective review 53 pediatric patients with a diagnosis of PPPD, and they reported that Common diagnoses in addition to PPPD included benign paroxysmal positional vertigo (64.2%), vestibular migraine (56.6%), and anxiety (28.3%) [51].

7. Vestibular function assessment for pediatric population

The children's vestibular function development is as follows. The vestibular function and specifically the vestibulo-ocular reflex is present at birth, although its time constants are about half of normal adult values at 2 months old [3]. The absence of a VOR by 10 months of age should be considered abnormal. The development of children's postural stability is that they first control the head, then the trunk, and finally the postural stability when standing. Regarding balance control, unlike adults, infants and children prefer visual inputs to vestibular information rather than somatosensory inputs in achieving postural equilibrium. At 3–6 years of age, children begin to use somatosensory information appropriately. In adolescents around the age of 15, the coordination of adult-like postural responses can be assumed due to complete maturation of the three sensory systems and the ability to solve intersensory conflict [52].

Currently, some vestibular tests are introduced as childhood vestibular function evaluation. The available vestibular function tests applied in children include cervical vestibular evoked myogenic potentials (cVEMP), ocular vestibular evoked myogenic potentials (oVEMP), video head impulse test (vHIT) and calorie test.

It is documented that rotatory chair, cVEMP and vHIT tests are feasible for children aged 0 ~ 2 years; for children aged 3 to 7 years, vHIT, cVEMP and oVEMP have satisfactory compliance; Children over 8 years old can cooperate well to complete vHIT, calorie test, cVEMP and oVEMP test. All these tests are well tolerated by children and relatively easy-to-use, and simple to operate. Additionally, it should be noted that the test procedure requires an individualized process, that is the protocol should be adjusted according to the condition of each subject [53].

Dhondt et al. conducted vestibular tests for 58 healthy children between 5 months and 6 years of age, and found that most subjects can complete the vestibular tests, the completion rate from high to low was cVEMP, oVEMP, vHIT, rotatory test and caloric test [54]. Similar result was demonstrated by Verrecchia et al., and they found that the best compliance was achieved for HIT (97.1%) and least for cVEMP (68.6%) in pediatric cochlear implants candidates [55].

Some causes may lead to a low compliance of vestibular test in children. For example, due to lack of attention or interest for the target or their gaze diversions, a naturally depressed vestibular function [56] and gaze fixation [57] may present in very young children (<6 months), so their HIT can result falsely pathological results. In VEMP, due to various procedural biases in VEMP recording, the risk for false pathological results is also common, because it is difficult to keep a stable and sustained neck muscle activation in unconstrained children [55].

vHIT is the most widely used tool for pediatric vestibular function assessment. In terms of the diagnostic value of vHIT, recent studies showed that the vHIT test is a sensitive and efficient vestibular test in the pediatric population [58, 59], although the sensitivity of vHIT may be lower than caloric test in vestibular dysfunction detection, particularly in the pediatric population [59]. Moreover, due to the low compliance of caloric test in young children, vHIT is selected to be a regular vestibular test for young children. Regarding balance tests, it is reported that children with unilateral vestibular impairment showed normal balance function, which indicates that vestibular compensation enables them to rely on vestibular input to keep balance. As a result, it is difficult to judge the extent of vestibular dysfunction by using balance tests alone [60].

8. Vestibular dysfunction in pediatric patients

Children with vestibular diseases can present with the same vestibular function abnormalities as adults who suffer from the same diseases. For example, pediatric patients with VM have higher values of gain compared to asymptomatic patients [61]. In addition, children with Meniere disease exhibit a significantly vestibular function declining sequence from the cochlea, to the saccule, utricle and semicircular canals [62].

Vestibular dysfunction may also occur in children affected with some auditory diseases but without vertigo symptoms. Children with SNHL can exhibit vestibular impairment, given the embryological and anatomical connection between the cochlea and vestibular end-organs and their shared sensory microstructure and genetics [63]. Another example is otitis media with effusion, previous studies revealed that approximately 30% of the children with OME have some degree of vestibular impairment documented with vestibular test [64, 65]. Moreover, the vestibular impairment among OME patients may be not severe. A study results showed that the mean vHIT gains and gain asymmetry values of pediatric with OME and dizziness and healthy children were comparable. However, covert saccades were observed in 57% of the patients with OME and dizziness, but none patients had overt saccades [66].

Some researchers have described vestibular hypofunction in children with cytomegalovirus infection, vestibular neuritis, complicated cholesteatoma, post traumatic vertigo, motion sickness and auditory neuropathy [67–73].

One hotpot of pediatric vestibular disorders is the evaluation of post-cochlear-implantation vestibular function. Recent evidence has demonstrated a relatively wide range of patients suffered from vestibular dysfunction after cochlear implantation [74–76], and the total equilibrium score was also significantly reduced in implanted children than the non-operative controls [77]. Different mechanisms have been proposed to explain this phenomenon, including electrical stimulation by the prosthesis, direct trauma following electrode placement, foreign body reaction or labyrinthitis, and endolymphatic hydrops [76, 78–80].

Author details

Wen Xie[1,2] and Maoli Duan[2*]

1 Department of Otolaryngology, Head and Neck Surgery, The Second Affiliated Hospital of Nanchang University, Nanchang, China

2 Division of Ear, Nose and Throat Diseases, Department of Clinical Science, Intervention and Technology, Karolinska Institutet and Department of Otolaryngology Head and Neck and Audiology and Neurotology, Karolinska University Hospital, Stockholm, Sweden

*Address all correspondence to: maoli.duan@ki.se

References

[1] Organization WH. Childhood Hearing Loss: Strategies for Prevention and Care. 1st ed. Geneva (Switzerland): World Health Organization; 2016. pp. 1-28

[2] Butcher E, Dezateux C, Cortina-Borja M, et al. Prevalence of permanent childhood hearing loss detected at the universal newborn hearing screen: Systematic review and meta-analysis. PLoS One. 2019;**14**(7):e0219600

[3] Bussé AML, Hoeve HLJ, Nasserinejad K, et al. Prevalence of permanent neonatal hearing impairment: Systematic review and bayesian meta-analysis. International Journal of Audiology. 2020;**59**(6):475-485

[4] Osei AO, Larnyo PA, Azaglo A, et al. Screening for hearing loss among school going children. International Journal of Pediatric Otorhinolaryngology. 2018;**111**:7-12

[5] Niemensivu R, Pyykkö I, Wiener-Vacher SR, et al. Vertigo and balance problems in children—An epidemiologic study in Finland. International Journal of Pediatric Otorhinolaryngology. 2006;**70**(2):259-265

[6] O'Reilly RC, Morlet T, Nicholas BD, et al. Prevalence of vestibular and balance disorders in children. Otology & Neurotology. 2010;**31**(9):1441-1444

[7] Bigelow RT, Semenov YR, Hoffman HJ, et al. Association between vertigo, cognitive and psychiatric conditions in us children: 2012 national health interview survey. International Journal of Pediatric Otorhinolaryngology. 2020;**130**:109802

[8] Lieu JEC, Kenna M, Anne S, et al. Hearing loss in children: A review. Journal of the American Medical Association. 2020;**324**(21):2195-2205

[9] Year 2007 position statement: Principles and guidelines for early hearing detection and intervention programs. Pediatrics. 2007;**120**(4):898-921

[10] Niu K, Brandström A, Skenbäck S, et al. Risk factors and etiology of childhood hearing loss: A cohort review of 296 subjects. Acta Oto-Laryngologica. 2020;**140**(8):668-674

[11] Kenneson A, Cannon MJ. Review and meta-analysis of the epidemiology of congenital cytomegalovirus (cmv) infection. Reviews in Medical Virology. 2007;**17**(4):253-276

[12] Boppana SB, Ross SA, Shimamura M, et al. Saliva polymerase-chain-reaction assay for cytomegalovirus screening in newborns. The New England Journal of Medicine. 2011;**364**(22):2111-2118

[13] Dollard SC, Grosse SD, Ross DS. New estimates of the prevalence of neurological and sensory sequelae and mortality associated with congenital cytomegalovirus infection. Reviews in Medical Virology. 2007;**17**(5):355-363

[14] Marsico C, Kimberlin DW. Congenital cytomegalovirus infection: Advances and challenges in diagnosis, prevention and treatment. Italian Journal of Pediatrics. 2017;**43**(1):38

[15] Dahle AJ, Fowler KB, Wright JD, et al. Longitudinal investigation of hearing disorders in children with congenital cytomegalovirus. Journal of the American Academy of Audiology. 2000;**11**(5):283-290

[16] Fowler KB, McCollister FP, Dahle AJ, et al. Progressive and fluctuating sensorineural hearing loss in children with asymptomatic congenital cytomegalovirus infection. The Journal of Pediatrics. 1997;**130**(4):624-630

[17] Korver AM, Smith RJ, Van Camp G, et al. Congenital hearing loss. Nature Reviews. Disease Primers. 2017;**3**:16094

[18] homepage Hhl. Posted January 25, 2020. Updated August 30, 2021. Available from: https://hereditaryhearingloss.org [Accessed: May 4, 2022]

[19] Kelsell DP, Dunlop J, Stevens HP, et al. Connexin 26 mutations in hereditary non-syndromic sensorineural deafness. Nature. 1997;**387**(6628):80-83

[20] Chang KW. Genetics of hearing loss—Nonsyndromic. Otolaryngologic Clinics of North America. 2015;**48**(6): 1063-1072

[21] Liu X, Xu L, Zhang S, et al. Epidemiological and genetic studies of congenital profound deafness in the general population of Sichuan, China. American Journal of Medical Genetics. 1994;**53**(2):192-195

[22] Smith RJ, Bale JF Jr, White KR. Sensorineural hearing loss in children. Lancet. 2005;**365**(9462):879-890

[23] Liu XZ, Angeli S, Ouyang XM, et al. Audiological and genetic features of the mtdna mutations. Acta Oto-Laryngologica. 2008;**128**(7):732-738

[24] Božanić Urbančič N, Battelino S, Tesovnik T, et al. The importance of early genetic diagnostics of hearing loss in children. Medicina (Kaunas, Lithuania). 2020;**56**(9):471

[25] Carey JC, Palumbos JC. Advances in the understanding of the genetic causes of hearing loss in children inform a rational approach to evaluation. Indian Journal of Pediatrics. 2016;**83**(10):1150-1156

[26] Kenna MA. Acquired hearing loss in children. Otolaryngologic Clinics of North America. 2015;**48**(6):933-953

[27] Tos M. Epidemiology and natural history of secretory otitis. The American Journal of Otology. 1984;**5**(6):459-462

[28] Organization WH. Newborn and Infant Hearing Screening: Current Issues and Guiding Principles. Geneva (Switzerland): WHO Press; 2009. Accessed 16 May 2022

[29] Ringger J, Holden K, McRedmond M. Clinical test batteries to diagnose hearing loss in infants and children: The cross-check principle. Otolaryngologic Clinics of North America. 2021;**54**(6):1143-1154

[30] Duan M, Xie W, Persson L, et al. Postnatal hearing loss: A study of children who passed neonatal teoae hearing screening bilaterally. Acta Oto-Laryngologica. 2022;**142**(1):61-66

[31] De Leenheer EM, Janssens S, Padalko E, et al. Etiological diagnosis in the hearing impaired newborn: Proposal of a flow chart. International Journal of Pediatric Otorhinolaryngology. 2011;**75**(1):27-32

[32] Litwin CM, Hill HR. Serologic and DNA-based testing for congenital and perinatal infections. The Pediatric Infectious Disease Journal. 1997;**16**(12):1166-1175

[33] Raymond M, Walker E, Dave I, et al. Genetic testing for congenital non-syndromic sensorineural hearing loss. International Journal of Pediatric Otorhinolaryngology. 2019;**124**:68-75

[34] Retterer K, Juusola J, Cho MT, et al. Clinical application of whole-exome sequencing across clinical indications. Genetics in Medicine. 2016;**18**(7):696-704

[35] Belcher R, Virgin F, Duis J, et al. Genetic and non-genetic workup for pediatric congenital hearing loss. Frontiers in Pediatrics. 2021;**9**:536730

[36] Sommen M, Wuyts W, Van Camp G. Molecular diagnostics for hereditary hearing loss in children. Expert Review of Molecular Diagnostics. 2017;**17**(8):751-760

[37] Sommen MVCG, Boudewyns A. Genetic and clinical diagnosis in non-syndromic hearing loss. Hearing, Balance and Communication. 2004;**11**(3):904-809

[38] Wang RY, Earl DL, Ruder RO, et al. Syndromic ear anomalies and renal ultrasounds. Pediatrics. 2001;**108**(2):E32

[39] Nikolopoulos TP, Lioumi D, Stamataki S, et al. Evidence-based overview of ophthalmic disorders in deaf children: A literature update. Otology & Neurotology. 2006;**27**(2 Suppl 1):S1-S24. discussion S20

[40] Konrádsson K, Magnusson M, Andréasson S. Perform vestibular test among all small deaf children! Early detection of usher syndrome improves the possibilities of communication in the event of later deaf-blindness. Läkartidningen. 1998;**95**(5):379-381

[41] Amorim AM, Ribeiro JC. Prevalence of pediatric vestibular disorders. Acta Médica Portuguesa. 2021;**34**(9):644-645

[42] Brodsky JR, Lipson S, Bhattacharyya N. Prevalence of pediatric dizziness and imbalance in the United States. Otolaryngology and Head and Neck Surgery. 2020;**162**(2):241-247

[43] Lima AF, Moreira FC, Menezes AS, et al. Vestibular disorders in the pediatric age: Retrospective analysis and review of the literature. Acta Médica Portuguesa. 2021;**34**(6):428-434

[44] Gedik-Soyuyuce O, Gence-Gumus Z, Ozdilek A, et al. Vestibular disorders in children: A retrospective analysis of vestibular function test findings. International Journal of Pediatric Otorhinolaryngology. 2021;**146**:110751

[45] Božanić Urbančič N, Vozel D, Urbančič J, et al. Unraveling the etiology of pediatric vertigo and dizziness: A tertiary pediatric center experience. Medicina (Kaunas, Lithuania). 2021;**57**(5):475

[46] Dodick DW. Migraine. Lancet. 2018;**391**(10127):1315-1330

[47] Gelfand AA. Episodic syndromes of childhood associated with migraine. Current Opinion in Neurology. 2018;**31**(3):281-285

[48] Wiener-Vacher SRQJ, Le Priol A. Contemporary concepts in pediatric vestibular assessment and management: Epidemiology of vestibular impairments in a pediatric population. Seminars in Hearing. 2018:229. hieme Medical Publishers

[49] van, de Berg R, Widdershoven J, Bisdorff A, et al. Vestibular migraine of childhood and recurrent vertigo of childhood: Diagnostic criteria consensus document of the committee for the classification of vestibular disorders of the bárány society and the international headache society. Journal of Vestibular Research. 2021;**31**(1):1-9

[50] Schwam ZG, Wana G. Pediatric Vestibular Disorders. Diagnosis and Treatment of Vestibular Disorders. Berlin/Heidelberg, Germany: Springer; 2019. pp. 353-361

[51] Wang A, Fleischman KM, Kawai K, et al. Persistent postural-perceptual dizziness in children and adolescents. Otology & Neurotology. 2021;**42**(8):e1093-e1100

[52] Cushing SL, Papsin BC. Special considerations for the pediatric patient. Advances in Oto-Rhino-Laryngology. 2019;**82**:134-142

[53] Janky KL, Rodriguez AI. Quantitative vestibular function testing in the pediatric population. Seminars in Hearing. 2018;**39**(3):257-274

[54] Dhondt C, Dhooge I, Maes L. Vestibular assessment in the pediatric population. The Laryngoscope. 2019;**129**(2):490-493

[55] Verrecchia L, Galle Barrett K, Karltorp E. The feasibility, validity and reliability of a child friendly vestibular assessment in infants and children candidates to cochlear implant. International Journal of Pediatric Otorhinolaryngology. 2020;**135**:110093

[56] Wiener-Vacher SR, Wiener SI. Video head impulse tests with a remote camera system: Normative values of semicircular canal vestibulo-ocular reflex gain in infants and children. Frontiers in Neurology. 2017;**8**:434

[57] Aring E, Grönlund MA, Hellström A, et al. Visual fixation development in children. Graefe's Archive for Clinical and Experimental Ophthalmology. 2007;**245**(11):1659-1665

[58] Hamilton SS, Zhou G, Brodsky JR. Video head impulse testing (vhit) in the pediatric population. International Journal of Pediatric Otorhinolaryngology. 2015;**79**(8):1283-1287

[59] Ross LM, Helminski JO. Test-retest and interrater reliability of the video head impulse test in the pediatric population. Otology & Neurotology. 2016;**37**(5):558-563

[60] Van Hecke R, Deconinck FJA, Wiersema JR, et al. Balanced growth project: A protocol of a single-Centre observational study on the involvement of the vestibular system in a child's motor and cognitive development. BMJ Open. 2021;**11**(6):e049165

[61] Rodríguez-Villalba R, Caballero-Borrego M, Villarraga V, et al. Vestibulo-ocular reflex assessed with video head impulse test in children with vestibular migraine: Our experience. International Journal of Pediatric Otorhinolaryngology. 2020;**137**:110161

[62] Wang C, Wu CH, Cheng PW, et al. Pediatric meniere's disease. International Journal of Pediatric Otorhinolaryngology. 2018;**105**:16-19

[63] Wrobel C, Zafeiriou MP, Moser T. Understanding and treating paediatric hearing impairment. eBioMedicine. 2021;**63**:103171

[64] Monsanto RDC, Kasemodel ALP, Tomaz A, et al. Current evidence of peripheral vestibular symptoms secondary to otitis media. Annals of Medicine. 2018;**50**(5):391-401

[65] Koyuncu M, Saka MM, Tanyeri Y, et al. Effects of otitis media with effusion on the vestibular system in children. Otolaryngology and Head and Neck Surgery. 1999;**120**(1):117-121

[66] Tozar M, Cömert E, Şencan Z, et al. Video head impulse test in children with otitis media with effusion and dizziness. International Journal of Pediatric Otorhinolaryngology. 2020;**129**:109783

[67] Dhondt C, Maes L, Oostra A, et al. Episodic vestibular symptoms in children

with a congenital cytomegalovirus infection: A case series. Otology & Neurotology. 2019;**40**(6):e636-e642

[68] Wiener-Vacher SR, Quarez J, Priol AL. Epidemiology of vestibular impairments in a pediatric population. Seminars in Hearing. 2018;**39**(3):229-242

[69] Zhou G, Goutos C, Lipson S, et al. Clinical significance of spontaneous nystagmus in pediatric patients. International Journal of Pediatric Otorhinolaryngology. 2018;**111**:103-107

[70] Lipson S, Wang A, Corcoran M, et al. Severe motion sickness in infants and children. European Journal of Paediatric Neurology. 2020;**28**:176-179

[71] Stahl MC, Otteson T. Systematic review on vestibular symptoms in patients with enlarged vestibular aqueducts. The Laryngoscope. 2022;**132**(4):873-880

[72] Pinninti S, Christy J, Almutairi A, et al. Vestibular, gaze, and balance disorders in asymptomatic congenital cytomegalovirus infection. Pediatrics. 2021;**147**(2):e20193945

[73] Hu J, Chen Z, Zhang Y, et al. Vestibular dysfunction in patients with auditory neuropathy detected by vestibular evoked myogenic potentials. Clinical Neurophysiology. 2020;**131**(7):1664-1671

[74] Krause E, Louza JP, Hempel JM, et al. Prevalence and characteristics of preoperative balance disorders in cochlear implant candidates. The Annals of Otology, Rhinology, and Laryngology. 2008;**117**(10):764-768

[75] Abramides PA, Bittar RS, Tsuji RK, et al. Caloric test as a predictor tool of postural control in ci users. Acta Oto-Laryngologica. 2015;**135**(7):685-691

[76] Buchman CA, Joy J, Hodges A, et al. Vestibular effects of cochlear implantation. Laryngoscope. 2004;**114**(10 Pt 2 Suppl 103):1-22

[77] Bayat A, Farhadi M, Emamdjomeh H, et al. Influence of cochlear implantation on balance function in pediatrics. The International Tinnitus Journal. 2020;**24**(1):xxx-xx

[78] Ibrahim I, da Silva SD, Segal B, et al. Effect of cochlear implant surgery on vestibular function: Meta-analysis study. Journal of Otolaryngology—Head & Neck Surgery. 2017;**46**(1):44

[79] Nordfalk KF, Rasmussen K, Hopp E, et al. Insertion depth in cochlear implantation and outcome in residual hearing and vestibular function. Ear and Hearing. 2016;**37**(2):e129-e137

[80] Bittar RSM, Sato ES, Ribeiro DJS, et al. Preoperative vestibular assessment protocol of cochlear implant surgery: An analytical descriptive study. Brazilian Journal of Otorhinolaryngology. 2017;**83**(5):530-535

Chapter 2

Evidence of a Neuroinflammatory Model of Tinnitus

Raheel Ahmed and Rumana Ahmed

Abstract

Emerging literature has highlighted the relationship between inflammatory and neuroinflammatory biomarkers and tinnitus. Neuroinflammation may help to explain the mechanisms underpinning hyperactivity in the cochlea, cochlear nucleus, inferior colliculus, medial geniculate body, and the auditory cortex in those with tinnitus. Glial activation and pro-inflammatory cytokines may cause excitatory-inhibitory synaptic imbalance. Advancing our understanding of these mechanisms may help elucidate the pathogenesis of tinnitus and lead to improvement in subtyping subjective tinnitus. The chapter explores our current understanding of the neuroinflammatory model within the context of the classical auditory pathway and what we can infer about the underlying mechanisms based on these studies.

Keywords: neuroinflammation, tinnitus, inflammation, biomarkers, platelets, neuroglia, microglia, hyperactivity, cytokines, genetics, synaptic plasticity, neuroinflammatory biomarkers

1. Introduction

Tinnitus is an auditory perception with no external stimulus. It often presents as a ringing or buzzing sound in one or both ears or in the head and can be intermittent. Tinnitus can be subjective or objective. Objective tinnitus can be categorized into subtypes based on known sound sources. These categories include neurological disorders (myoclonus), vascular disorders, temporomandibular disorders (TMD), and patulous Eustachian tube. Palatal myoclonus is a series of sporadic muscle contractions by the tensor veli palatini muscle in the soft palate. The condition can be categorized as either essential or symptomatic through symptomatic manifestation or the presence of physical lesions in the cerebellum or brainstem [1]. Stapedial myoclonus describes similar muscle contractions of the tensor tympani and the stapedial muscles leading to the subject hearing a constant clicking sound from the vibration of the tympanic membrane [2]. Some case reports suggest individuals with TMD and tinnitus can modulate their tinnitus through head or jaw movements. The pathogenesis for tinnitus remains unclear, but tinnitus can be alleviated by treating the TMD [3].

Patulous Eustachian tube (PET) often presents with aural fullness, autophony, and tinnitus [4]. PET is caused when the Eustachian tube fails to close. Vascular disorders cause pulsatile tinnitus. This occurs when the sound of blood flow becomes audible due to increased blood pressure disrupting laminar flow [5]. Compression of the ipsilateral

Subjective tinnitus	Objective tinnitus
Ototoxicity	Patulous Eustachian tube
Noise exposure	Neurological disorders
Traumatic event	Vascular disorders
Ménière's disease	Superior semicircular canal dehiscence
Hearing loss	

Table 1.
Known causes of subjective and objective tinnitus.

internal jugular vein may accentuate or attenuate the sound of pulsatile tinnitus, depending on whether it is arterial or venous in etiology [6]. Pulsatile tinnitus, presenting with or without asymmetrical hearing loss, is regarded as a criterion for neuroimaging leading to a possible acoustic neuroma diagnosis, which may require surgical intervention [7, 8]. Pulsatile tinnitus is also a symptom of semicircular canal dehiscence alongside autophony, similarly to PET [9]. **Table 1** shows a list of causes of subjective and objective tinnitus.

2. Possible subtypes of subjective tinnitus

The term "tinnitus," on its own, typically refers to subjective tinnitus, which is a perceptual phenomenon with no physical counterpart or means to hear the sound by auscultation [10]. Subjective tinnitus can be idiopathic and can present as any type of sound, it can last from seconds to being constant. Subjective tinnitus is usually idiopathic but can present with a number of inflammatory diseases, one of such being Ménière's disease. Low-frequency narrow band tinnitus noise can be one of the earliest symptoms of Ménière's disease, which worsens in later stages, often becoming more intense before an episode of vertigo [10]. Cisplatin-based chemotherapy and many ototoxic medications can result in the development of subjective tinnitus, though the mechanisms underpinning this relationship remain unknown [11].

Subtyping tinnitus may be important for understanding tinnitus etiology and developing targeted treatments for each subtype, however, the rarity of subtypes (based on presentation) makes it difficult to conduct large-scale studies with representative samples. For example, "typewriter tinnitus" is a type of intermittent staccato-like tinnitus sound that has been thought to be related to vascular compression based on case-based neuroimaging and its response to the anticonvulsant carbamazepine [12]. However, there were only 12 cases of "typewriter tinnitus" recorded.

Subjective tinnitus is correlated with excitatory-inhibitory synaptic imbalance leading to hyperactivity in the auditory pathway; however, the cause of this balance has remained the subject of debate [13–15]. Recent studies indicate this process is underpinned by neuroinflammation through pro-inflammatory cytokines. Markers of this inflammation serve as potential biomarkers for the development of subtypes of subjective tinnitus [16, 17].

3. The current neuroinflammatory model of tinnitus

The synaptic connection between two neurons is strengthened by the firing of the presynaptic neuron shortly before the postsynaptic neuron, and this is known as

Hebbian plasticity. Conversely, anti-Hebbian plasticity is when the neurons fire out of sync or at the same time. The former leads to long-term potentiation (hyperactivity) and the latter leads to long-term depression; it is this temporal relationship in neuronal firing, which is involved in spike-timing-dependent plasticity (STDP) [18]. Changes in STDP and an increased spontaneous firing rate (SFR) are referred to as hyperactivity in the auditory pathway.

The neuroinflammatory model of tinnitus is still in its infancy with emerging literature limited to animal studies. The following sections will explore our current understanding of the neuroinflammatory model within the context of the classical auditory pathway and what we can infer about the underlying mechanisms based on these studies. Cytokines, microglia, and activated platelets all of these had documented associations with tinnitus, which could pave the way for reliable inflammatory biomarkers of tinnitus.

Short-term noise exposure can lead to a temporary hearing loss, whereas repeated or long-term noise exposure can lead to a permanent hearing loss, both of which are often accompanied by tinnitus. Similarly, the amount of ototoxic drug exposure can lead to temporary or permanent hearing loss and tinnitus [19]. Noise-induced hearing loss is caused by damage to inner and outer hair cells in the cochlea by acute noise exposure, the hearing loss is typically high-frequency and often presents with a high-pitch tinnitus sound [20]. Emotional and physical trauma can also contribute to tinnitus. There is a higher prevalence of tinnitus in individuals with post-traumatic stress disorder than in those working in noisy environments [20]. Many tinnitus treatments focus on stress management with the aim to reduce a tinnitus sufferer's levels of anxiety or distress, this helps alleviate tinnitus itself, or its negative effects on one's mental state [21].

In human populations, several non-auditory conditions, such as depression, stress, and traumatic brain injury, are risk factors for tinnitus [22]. These same conditions promote pro-inflammatory cytokine production in cerebrospinal fluid and contribute to neuroinflammation [17]. Genetic studies investigating single nucleotide polymorphisms have found associations between alleles contributing toward cytokine expression and susceptibility to develop noise-induced tinnitus. The frequency of the genotype for IL1α −889 C > T was found to be significantly associated with tinnitus in the elderly with a history of occupational noise exposure [23]. IL6 −174 G > C allele and TNFα −308 G > A allele frequency have been shown to be significantly associated with tinnitus in the elderly with a history of occupational noise exposure [24, 25].

Microglia may also play a role in neuroplasticity, beyond being simple scavengers that monitor and phagocytose waste products after neurodegeneration [26]. Microglia also produce pro-inflammatory cytokines, reactive oxygen species, and chemokines [27] as well as playing a role in neural maturation, aging and neuroplasticity, their pro-inflammatory cytokines regulate the function of neurons in synaptic plasticity [17]. A rodent study by Wang et al. [16] demonstrated neuroinflammatory events in the auditory cortex, following noise exposure. The study found microglial activation led to tumor necrosis factor-alpha (TNF-α) production and TNF-α further activated microglia, this feedback loop leads to an excitatory-inhibitory imbalance, which could be a cause of noise-induced tinnitus in the primary auditory cortex [13]. Following acoustic trauma, microglia upregulate TNF-α and IL-1β (interleukin-1 beta) cytokines in the cochlear nucleus on a much larger scale than in the auditory cortex [28]. This process of glial activation in neuroinflammation may inadvertently contribute to the pathogenesis of tinnitus, while trying to stabilize neuronal activity in the auditory pathway.

3.1 Tinnitus induction methods

Recent studies investigating tinnitus in animal models have typically used salicylate to induce tinnitus or noise exposure. The studies then measure their performance on the gap-prepulse inhibition of the acoustic startle reflex (GPIAS) to determine whether or not tinnitus is present [29]. The GPIAS paradigm relies on animals with tinnitus failing to elicit an acoustic startle response – a defensive reflex in response to loud noise. A silent gap in a continuous noise can inhibit this reflex in animals but the inability to perceive this gap due to tinnitus leads to the reflex being elicited [30].

4. In the context of the classical auditory pathway

4.1 The cochlea and cochlear nucleus

Roberts [19] proposes maladaptive plasticity within the auditory system as a reason for the development of tinnitus following noise-induced hearing loss. This phenomenon is supposedly due to homeostatic neuroplastic changes in neuronal firing leading to increased spontaneous activity in the auditory pathway to compensate for reduced input from the cochlea due to inner hair cell damage.

Martel et al. [31] suggest sodium salicylate increases SFRs and alters STDP through activating N-methyl-D-aspartate (NMDA) receptors, leading to tinnitus, as shown in **Figure 1** [32]. Ralli et al. [33] found that memantine, which acts as a non-competitive inhibitor of the NMDA receptor in the cochlea, was effective at reducing salicylate-induced tinnitus in rats but concluded that the side effects of consuming the dose required would outweigh the benefits. Salicylate-induced tinnitus may also be generated by an increase in the SFR in fusiform cells in the dorsal cochlear nucleus (DCN) as well as a change in STDP due to reduced auditory input from the cochlea [22].

It is this change from regular spiking to bursting activity in DCN fusiform cells that may underpin both noise-induced and salicylate-induced tinnitus in animal models [31, 34]. However, this is only true in spontaneous auditory nerve activity when high doses of sodium salicylate are used; moderate doses are capable of inducing tinnitus with no significant change in spontaneous neuronal firing [35]. Greater doses of salicylate are known to have more severe and irreversible effects on the auditory system [36]. Wu et al. [37] propose that noise-induced tinnitus also leads to increased parallel fiber excitation in DCN fusiform cells leading to an increase in SFRs. A reduction in inhibitory synapses on these DCN fusiform cells leads to burst firing and thus hyper-excitation. Variations in NMDA receptor expression across parallel fiber synapses on DCN and cartwheel cells may account for the differences in their Hebbian and anti-Hebbian plasticity, respectively [34].

Cartwheel cells are interneurons that release gamma-aminobutyric acid (GABA) and glycine – two inhibitory neurotransmitters, following noise exposure they are thought to reduce their activity. This downregulation at GABAergic and glycinergic synapses causes hyper-excitation in the fusiform cells of the DCN [34, 38].

Brozoski and Bauer [39] found that weeks after cochlear nucleus ablation, noise-induced tinnitus remained the same in rats; however, the DCN was considered ablated in the study even in cases where as much as 40% of it remained unaffected, as highlighted by Manzoor et al. [40]. Hyperactivity in the remaining DCN could still have been the cause of the noise-induced tinnitus in this case.

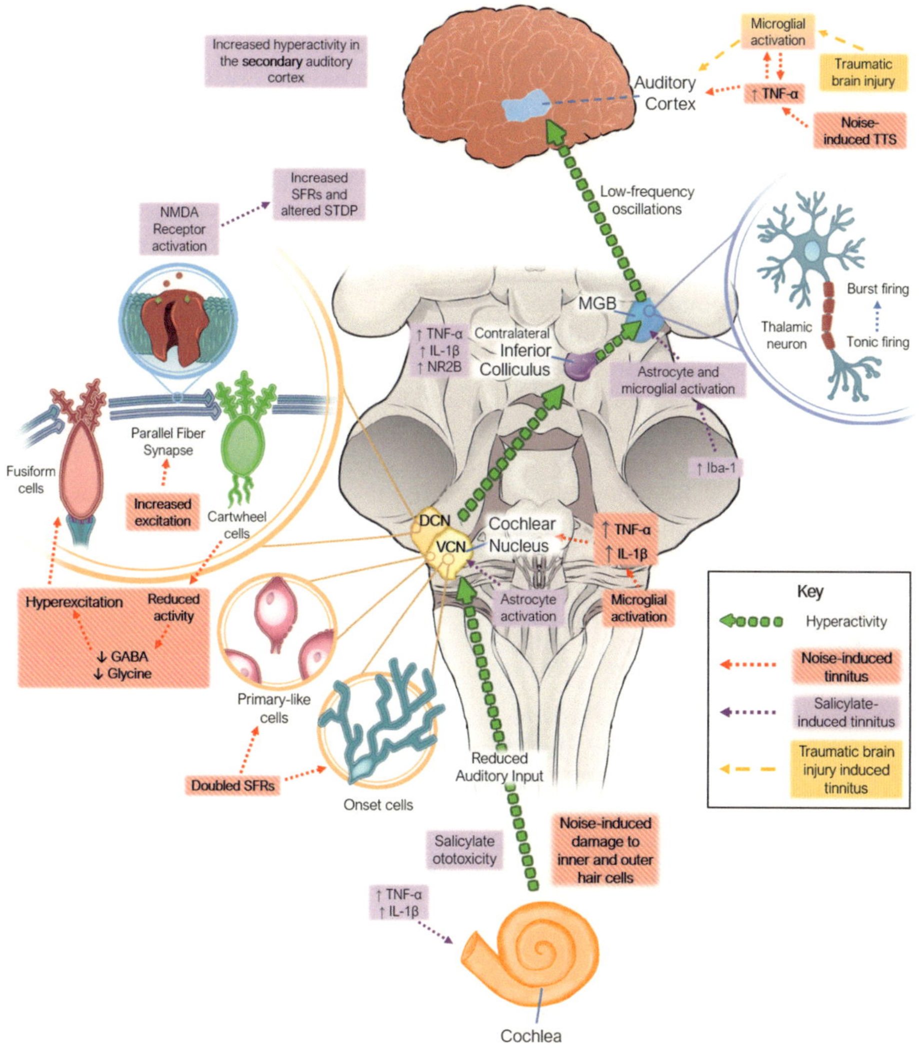

Figure 1.
The current neuroinflammatory model of tinnitus in the context of the classical auditory pathway. The figure shows theoretical causes and effects of hyperactivity in the cochlea, cochlear nucleus, inferior colliculus, medial geniculate body, and auditory cortex, based on findings in the current literature.

Vogler et al. [41] found that on average SFRs in the ventral cochlear nucleus (VCN) doubled in animals with noise-induced tinnitus, most significantly in primary-like and onset cells. Though many studies have explored DCN ablation when monitoring tinnitus in animal models [39, 40, 42], very few have examined hyperactivity in the primary-like cells and onset cells in the VCN and the inferior colliculus, which may sustain tinnitus post-ablation [41].

4.2 Inferior colliculus

Following acoustic trauma, hyperactivity in the inferior colliculus originates from activity in the afferent neurons in the cochlear contralateral to it, however, this dependency on the cochlea lessens the longer the hyperactivity remains in the cochlea [43]. This was demonstrated by [44] who performed cochlear ablation 2 weeks after acoustic trauma and found reduced hyperactivity, whereas in [45] where the same procedure was performed for 12 weeks after the acoustic trauma, found no significant difference in hyperactivity. Hyperactivity in the inferior colliculus may originate from the DCN or be an independent process altogether. Manzoor et al. [40] found that DCN ablation significantly reduced inferior colliculus hyperactivity in hamsters; however, ablation was performed 3 weeks after the development of noise-induced tinnitus. Though hyperactivity in the inferior colliculus likely originates from hyperactivity in the DCN [34], it is possible that hyperactivity in the inferior colliculus could to become endogenous given enough time after the onset of tinnitus [19].

Salicylate-induced tinnitus is known to lead to hyperactivity in the inferior colliculus and the secondary auditory cortex [36]. Tinnitus severity is correlated with an increase in TNF-α [46]. Measuring mRNA expression in mice with salicylate-induced tinnitus, Hwang et al. [47] found that TNF-α and IL-1β were significantly increased in the cochlea and the inferior colliculus as well as NMDA subtype 2B (NR2B) gene expression suggesting NMDA receptor action, which may be involved in long term potentiation leading to hyperactivity [35].

4.3 Medial geniculate body

The medial geniculate body is a known intermediary between the auditory cortex and the inferior colliculus in the classical auditory pathway; however, its role in tinnitus has not been well-examined [48]. Roberts [19] suggests following hyperactivity in the inferior colliculus, thalamic neurons switch from tonal firing to burst firing in the medial geniculate body. This change is caused by membrane hyperpolarization, which activates calcium channels causing thalamic neurons to carry less well-defined nonlinear inputs [48]. This may lead to low-frequency oscillations propagating to the auditory cortex [19].

Iba-1 (ionized calcium-binding adapter protein-1) expression can be used as a marker for increased microglial activation. Xia et al. [15] found Iba-1 was upregulated in the medial geniculate body and the primary auditory cortex in rats, evidencing microglial and astrocyte activation in salicylate-induced tinnitus [49]. The primary auditory cortex also showed increased IL-1β expression in its mRNA. IL-1β alongside other pro-inflammatory cytokines can regulate the excitatory-inhibitory balance through interactions with receptors on neuroglial cells [15].

4.4 Auditory cortex

Deng et al. [50] found greater microglial activation in the auditory cortex of rodents when subjected to 86 dB SPL noise at 8 kHz, following the intracerebroventricular infusion of TNF-α. This also impaired gap detection and prepulse inhibition that suggest the development of tinnitus. The same microglial activation was not present when subjected to the noise alone or when having received the TNF-α infusion alone. Similarly, Basura et al. [51] found stimulus timing-dependent responses followed anti-Hebbian timing rules in the primary auditory cortex of guinea pigs subjected to noise exposure, however, only those who developed tinnitus showed an increase in SFRs. Blast-induced traumatic brain injury results in microglial activation through an alternative pathway from acoustic trauma, one which is possibly independent of TNF-α interaction [14, 16]. Salicylate ototoxicity also leads to increased SFRs in the secondary auditory cortex [52].

Noise-induced hearing loss decreases activity at GABAergic synapses and increases activity at glutamatergic synapses in the auditory cortex, leading to an excitatory-inhibitory imbalance [53]. This may lead to spontaneous synchronous neuronal firing, which would cause long-term potentiation in the auditory cortex inducing tinnitus following acoustic trauma.

5. Peripheral inflammation

Peripheral inflammation and an increase in pro-inflammatory cytokines, such as TNF-α, can lead to neuroinflammatory processes in the brain [54]. In the past 30 years, it has become apparent that platelets are involved in more than just thrombocytosis in vascular injuries, despite this, little remains understood about their cytokine interactions and their role in neuroinflammation [55]. A meta-analysis by Ahmed et al. [56] synthesized data from six studies including 451 tinnitus sufferers and 367 controls, and found mean platelet volume (MPV) was significantly increased in populations with tinnitus, including in normal hearing populations. This suggests greater platelet activation in the tinnitus population and may serve as an easy-to-obtain and inexpensive biomarker of tinnitus [57, 58]. However, further research in this area must prioritize a well-reported methodology including the type of hematology analyzer used and the precise means through which the samples were collected. Additionally, further research must exclude individuals with existing inflammatory pathology as recommended in [56]. By reproducing the association with better documentation and improved methodology, we can better understand the exact mechanisms that underpin MPV as a candidate biomarker of subjective tinnitus and its relationship with neuroinflammatory processes.

6. Current limitations and further research

The meta-analysis by Ahmed et al. [56] used only a human population to demonstrate an increase in MPV in people with tinnitus compared to controls without tinnitus. The current literature examining cytokine interactions in the auditory pathway has primarily used animal studies. This is because current techniques for measuring neural activity in the human brain lack the cellular resolution to pinpoint the exact structures involved in tinnitus [59]. Guinea pigs and rodents are likely to be used since the human cochlear nucleus is cellularly similar to the rodent cochlear nucleus [60]. The GPIAS is commonly used to determine the presence of tinnitus in animals; however, the GPIAS has not been proven to be a valid measure of tinnitus in humans [29]. It is also not possible to distinguish between subtypes of subjective tinnitus based on the presentation in animals [48].

One limitation of this model that has not been discussed in the literature thus far is the relationship between the neuroinflammatory model and hearing loss or stress. Hyperactivity in the DCN, for example, has been shown to be affected by attentional and emotional responses just as tinnitus is [61]. Studies thus far do not seem to define the direction of this relationship. McKenna et al. [62] suggest that those without tinnitus have habituated to spontaneous neuronal firing but tinnitus occurs due to brief lapses in the ability to filter out these sounds. Those who become overly conscious and aware of these phantom sounds may then focus on this triggering a "fight or flight" response impeding their ability to filter out the sounds. It is this feedback loop that may lead to greater stress, which in turn increases neuroinflammation. A systematic review by Calcia et al. [63] found psychosocial stressors lead to microglial activation in the hippocampus, prefrontal cortex, and possibly other regions of the brain [64]. Deng et al. [50] overcame this limitation by comparing three conditions, one with the infusion of TNF-α, second with noise exposure, and the third with both. It was only in the lattermost condition where microglial activation occurred suggesting a causal relationship between noise-induced tinnitus and neuroinflammation.

The role of the VCN in leading to hyperactivity in the contralateral inferior colliculus and the role of the medial geniculate body require further investigation as the current literature on this subject is sparse. Future studies may wish to reexamine the positive feedback loop between microglia activation and TNF-α expression in the auditory cortex, which was observed by Wang et al. [16]. Further studies examining the association between MPV and tinnitus should work toward developing a more homogenous standardized methodology to recreate current findings [65].

Conflict of interest

The authors declare no conflict of interest.

Author details

Raheel Ahmed[1]* and Rumana Ahmed[2]

1 Liverpool University Hospitals NHS Foundation Trust, Liverpool, United Kingdom

2 Independent Scientist, United Kingdom, England

*Address all correspondence to: raheel.swanseauniversity@gmail.com

References

[1] Jankovic J, Mazziotta JC, Pomeroy SL, Newman NJ, editors. Bradley and Daroff's Neurology in Clinical Practice. Philadelphia (US): Elsevier; 2022

[2] Brigo F, Storti M, Lochner P, Nardone R. Transitory stapedial myoclonus in a patient with benign fasciculation syndrome. The Journal of Laryngology and Otology. 2013;**127**(6):605-606

[3] Vielsmeier V, Strutz J, Kleinjung T, Schecklmann M, Kreuzer PM, Landgrebe M, et al. Temporomandibular joint disorder complaints in tinnitus: Further hints for a putative tinnitus subtype. PLoS One. 2012;7(6):e38887

[4] Chari DA, Limb CJ. Tinnitus. Medical Clinics. 2018;**102**(6):1081-1093

[5] Hofmann E, Behr R, Neumann-Haefelin T, Schwager K. Pulsatile tinnitus: Imaging and differential diagnosis. Deutsches Ärzteblatt International. 2013 Jun;**110**(26):451

[6] Trivelato FP, Araújo JF, dos Santos SR, Rezende MT, Ulhôa AC, Castro GD. Endovascular treatment of pulsatile tinnitus associated with transverse sigmoid sinus aneurysms and jugular bulb anomalies. Interventional Neuroradiology. 2015;**21**(4):548-551

[7] NICE, 1.3 Investigation using MRI [Internet]. 2018. Available from: https://www.nice.org.uk/guidance/ng98/resources/hearing-loss-in-adults-assessment-and-management-pdf-1837761878725 [Accessed: March 15, 2022]

[8] Yew KS. Diagnostic approach to patients with tinnitus. American Family Physician. 2014;**89**(2):106-113

[9] Ward BK, Carey JP, Minor LB. Superior canal dehiscence syndrome: Lessons from the first 20 years. Frontiers in Neurology. 2017;**8**:177

[10] Perez-Carpena P, Lopez-Escamez JA. Current understanding and clinical management of Meniere's disease: a systematic review. In: Seminars in neurology. Thieme Medical Publishers. 2020 Feb;**40**(01):138-150

[11] El Charif O, Mapes B, Trendowski MR, Wheeler HE, Wing C, Dinh PC, et al. Clinical and genome-wide analysis of cisplatin-induced tinnitus implicates novel ototoxic mechanisms. Clinical Cancer Research. 2019;**25**(13):4104-4116

[12] Nam EC, Handzel O, Levine RA. Carbamazepine responsive typewriter tinnitus from basilar invagination. Journal of Neurology, Neurosurgery and Psychiatry. 2010;**81**(4):456-458

[13] Graeber MB, Li W, Rodriguez ML. Role of microglia in CNS inflammation. FEBS Letters. 2011;**585**(23):3798-3805

[14] Wang W, Zinsmaier AK, Firestone E, Lin R, Yatskievych TA, Yang S, et al. Blocking tumor necrosis factor-alpha expression prevents blast-induced excitatory/inhibitory synaptic imbalance and parvalbumin-positive interneuron loss in the hippocampus. Journal of Neurotrauma. 2018;**35**(19):2306-2316

[15] Xia C, Yin M, Wu C, Ji Y, Zhou Y. Neuroglial activation in the auditory cortex and medial geniculate body of salicylate-induced tinnitus rats. American Journal of Translational Research. 2020;**12**(10):6043

[16] Wang W, Zhang LS, Zinsmaier AK, Patterson G, Leptich EJ, Shoemaker SL,

et al. Neuroinflammation mediates noise-induced synaptic imbalance and tinnitus in rodent models. PLoS Biology. 2019;**17**(6):e3000307

[17] Shulman A, Wang W, Luo H, Bao S, Searchfield G, Zhang J. Neuroinflammation and Tinnitus. The Behavioral Neuroscience of Tinnitus. (Current Topics in Behavioral Neurosciences). 2021;**5**:161-174

[18] Caporale N, Dan Y. Spike timing–dependent plasticity: A Hebbian learning rule. Annual Review of Neuroscience. 2008;**31**:25-46

[19] Roberts LE. Neural plasticity and its initiating conditions in tinnitus. HNO. 2018;**66**(3):172-178

[20] Kreuzer PM, Landgrebe M, Vielsmeier V, Kleinjung T, De Ridder D, Langguth B. Trauma-associated tinnitus. The Journal of Head Trauma Rehabilitation. 2014;**29**(5):432-442

[21] Jun HJ, Park MK. Cognitive behavioral therapy for tinnitus: Evidence and efficacy. Korean Journal of Audiology. 2013;**17**(3):101

[22] Shore SE, Roberts LE, Langguth B. Maladaptive plasticity in tinnitus—triggers, mechanisms and treatment. Nature Reviews Neurology. 2016;**12**(3):150-160

[23] de Moraes Marchiori LL, Doi MY, de Moraes MG, de Souza GV, Poli-Frederico RC, de Almeida Ciquinato DS. Interleukin-1 alpha gene polymorphism (IL-1α) and susceptibility to tinnitus in the elderly. Noise and Health. 2019;**21**(99):77

[24] Doi MY, Dias AC, Poly-Frederico RC, Maria MG, de Oliveira MN, de Moraes Marchiori LL. Association between polymorphism of interleukin-6 in the region-174G/C and tinnitus in the elderly with a history of occupational noise exposure. Noise and Health. 2015;**17**(79):406

[25] Marchiori LL, Dias AC, Gonçalvez AS, Poly-Frederico RC, Doi MY. Association between polymorphism of tumor necrosis factor alpha (tnfα) in the region– 308 g/a with tinnitus in the elderly with a history of occupational noise exposure. Noise and Health. 2018;**20**(93):37

[26] Baizer JS, Wong KM, Manohar S, Hayes SH, Ding D, Dingman R, et al. Effects of acoustic trauma on the auditory system of the rat: The role of microglia. Neuroscience. 2015;**303**:299-311

[27] Wilkinson K, El Khoury J. Microglial scavenger receptors and their roles in the pathogenesis of Alzheimer's disease. International Journal of Alzheimer's Disease. 2012;**2012**

[28] Fuentes-Santamaría V, Alvarado JC, Melgar-Rojas P, Gabaldón-Ull MC, Miller JM, Juiz JM. The role of glia in the peripheral and central auditory system following noise overexposure: Contribution of TNF-α and IL-1β to the pathogenesis of hearing loss. Frontiers in Neuroanatomy. 2017;**11**:9

[29] Boyen K, Başkent D, van Dijk P. The gap detection test: Can it be used to diagnose tinnitus? Ear and hearing. 2015;**36**(4):e138

[30] Turner JG, Brozoski TJ, Bauer CA, Parrish JL, Myers K, Hughes LF, et al. Gap detection deficits in rats with tinnitus: A potential novel screening tool. Behavioral Neuroscience. 2006;**120**(1):188

[31] Martel DT, Pardo-Garcia TR, Shore SE. Dorsal cochlear nucleus fusiform-cell plasticity is altered in salicylate-induced tinnitus. Neuroscience. 2019;**407**:170-181

[32] Hwang JH, Chen JC, Chan YC. Effects of C-phycocyanin and Spirulina on salicylate-induced tinnitus, expression of NMDA receptor and inflammatory genes. PLoS One. 2013;**8**(3):e58215

[33] Ralli M, Troiani D, Podda MV, Paciello F, Eramo SL, De Corso E, et al. The effect of the NMDA channel blocker memantine on salicylate-induced tinnitus in rats. Acta Otorhinolaryngologica Italica. 2014;**34**(3):198

[34] Wu C, Stefanescu RA, Martel DT, Shore SE. Tinnitus: Maladaptive auditory–somatosensory plasticity. Hearing Research. 2016;**334**:20-29

[35] Stolzberg D, Salvi RJ, Allman BL. Salicylate toxicity model of tinnitus. Frontiers in Systems Neuroscience. 2012;**6**:28

[36] Cazals Y. Auditory sensori-neural alterations induced by salicylate. Progress in Neurobiology. 2000;**62**(6):583-631

[37] Wu C, Martel DT, Shore SE. Increased synchrony and bursting of dorsal cochlear nucleus fusiform cells correlate with tinnitus. Journal of Neuroscience. 2016;**36**(6):2068-2073

[38] Wang H, Brozoski TJ, Turner JG, Ling L, Parrish JL, Hughes LF, et al. Plasticity at glycinergic synapses in dorsal cochlear nucleus of rats with behavioral evidence of tinnitus. Neuroscience. 2009;**164**(2):747-759

[39] Brozoski TJ, Bauer CA. The effect of dorsal cochlear nucleus ablation on tinnitus in rats. Hearing Research. 2005;**206**(1-2):227-236

[40] Manzoor NF, Licari FG, Klapchar M, Elkin RL, Gao Y, Chen G, et al. Noise-induced hyperactivity in the inferior colliculus: Its relationship with hyperactivity in the dorsal cochlear nucleus. Journal of Neurophysiology. 2012;**108**(4):976-988

[41] Vogler DP, Robertson D, Mulders WH. Hyperactivity in the ventral cochlear nucleus after cochlear trauma. Journal of Neuroscience. 2011;**31**(18):6639-6645

[42] Brozoski TJ, Wisner KW, Sybert LT, Bauer CA. Bilateral dorsal cochlear nucleus lesions prevent acoustic-trauma induced tinnitus in an animal model. Journal of the Association for Research in Otolaryngology. 2012;**13**(1):55-66

[43] Robertson D, Bester C, Vogler D, Mulders WH. Spontaneous hyperactivity in the auditory midbrain: Relationship to afferent input. Hearing Research. 2013;**295**:124-129

[44] Mulders WH, Robertson D. Hyperactivity in the auditory midbrain after acoustic trauma: Dependence on cochlear activity. Neuroscience. 2009;**164**(2):733-746

[45] Mulders WH, Robertson D. Progressive centralization of midbrain hyperactivity after acoustic trauma. Neuroscience. 2011;**192**:753-760

[46] Weber C, Arck P, Mazurek B, Klapp BF. Impact of a relaxation training on psychometric and immunologic parameters in tinnitus sufferers. Journal of Psychosomatic Research. 2002;**52**(1):29-33

[47] Hwang JH, Chen JC, Yang SY, Wang MF, Chan YC. Expression of tumor necrosis factor-α and interleukin-1β genes in the cochlea and inferior colliculus in salicylate-induced tinnitus. Journal of Neuroinflammation. 2011;**8**(1):1-6

[48] Brinkmann P, Kotz SA, Smit JV, Janssen ML, Schwartze M. Auditory thalamus dysfunction and pathophysiology in tinnitus: A predictive network hypothesis. Brain Structure and Function. 2021;**226**(6):1659-1676

[49] Hovens IB, Nyakas C, Schoemaker RG. A novel method for evaluating microglial activation using ionized calcium-binding adaptor protein-1 staining: Cell body to cell size ratio. Neuroimmunology and Neuroinflammation. 2014;**1**:82-88

[50] Deng D, Wang W, Bao S. Diffusible tumor necrosis factor-alpha (TNF-α) promotes noise-induced parvalbumin-positive (PV+) neuron loss and auditory processing impairments. Frontiers in Neuroscience. 2020;**1065**

[51] Basura GJ, Koehler SD, Shore SE. Bimodal stimulus timing-dependent plasticity in primary auditory cortex is altered after noise exposure with and without tinnitus. Journal of Neurophysiology. 2015;**114**(6):3064-3075

[52] Chen GD, Stolzberg D, Lobarinas E, Sun W, Ding D, Salvi R. Salicylate-induced cochlear impairments, cortical hyperactivity and re-tuning, and tinnitus. Hearing research. 2013;**295**:100-113

[53] Browne CJ, Morley JW, Parsons CH. Tracking the expression of excitatory and inhibitory neurotransmission-related proteins and neuroplasticity markers after noise induced hearing loss. PLoS One. 2012;**7**(3):e33272

[54] Yang G, Parkhurst CN, Hayes S, Gan WB. Peripheral elevation of TNF-α leads to early synaptic abnormalities in the mouse somatosensory cortex in experimental autoimmune encephalomyelitis. Proceedings of the National Academy of Sciences. 2013;**110**(25):10306-10311

[55] Horstman LL, Jy W, Ahn YS, Zivadinov R, Maghzi AH, Etemadifar M, et al. Role of platelets in neuroinflammation: A wide-angle perspective. Journal of Neuro-inflammation. 2010 Dec;7(1):1-22

[56] Ahmed R, Shadis A, Ahmed R. Potential inflammatory biomarkers for tinnitus in platelets and leukocytes: A critical scoping review and meta-analysis. International Journal of Audiology. 2021:1-2

[57] Adhya Z, Borozdenkova S, Karim MY. The role of cytokines as biomarkers in systemic lupus erythematosus and lupus nephritis. Nephrology Dialysis Transplantation. 2011;**26**(10):3273-3280

[58] Kisacik B, Tufan A, Kalyoncu U, Karadag O, Akdogan A, Ozturk MA, et al. Mean platelet volume (MPV) as an inflammatory marker in ankylosing spondylitis and rheumatoid arthritis. Joint, Bone, Spine. 2008;**75**(3):291-294

[59] Clayton KK, Koops EA. An auditory phantom percept that does not impair external sound perception. Journal of Neuroscience. 2021;**41**(8):1622-1624

[60] Wagoner JL, Kulesza RJ Jr. Topographical and cellular distribution of perineuronal nets in the human cochlear nucleus. Hearing Research. 2009;**254**(1-2):42-53

[61] Kaltenbach JA. The dorsal cochlear nucleus as a participant in the auditory, attentional and emotional components of tinnitus. Hearing Research. 2006;**216**:224-234

[62] McKenna L, Baguley D, McFerran D. Living with Tinnitus and Hyperacusis: New Edition. London (UK): Sheldon press; 2021 Sep 30

[63] Calcia MA, Bonsall DR, Bloomfield PS, Selvaraj S, Barichello T, Howes OD. Stress and neuroinflammation: A systematic review of the effects of

stress on microglia and the implications for mental illness. Psychopharmacology. 2016;**233**(9):1637-1650

[64] Munhoz CD, Garcia-Bueno B, Madrigal JL, Lepsch LB, Scavone C, Leza JC. Stress-induced neuroinflammation: Mechanisms and new pharmacological targets. Brazilian Journal of Medical and Biological Research. 2008;**41**(12):1037-1046

[65] Haider HF, Hoare DJ, Ribeiro SF, Ribeiro D, Caria H, Trigueiros N, et al. Evidence for biological markers of tinnitus: A systematic review. Progress in Brain Research. 2021;**262**:345-398

Chapter 3

Signal Transmission by Auditory and Vestibular Hair Cells

Sergio Masetto, Paolo Spaiardi and Stuart J. Johnson

Abstract

We interact with the world around us by sensing a vast array of inputs and translating them into signals that can be interpreted by the brain. We have evolved many sensory receptors, each uniquely specialised to detect diverse stimuli. The hair cells are sensory receptors, initially developed to provide a sense of body position and movement, but later adapted to sense minute pressure waves in the environment that are perceived as sounds. As such, hair cells bestow a sense of hearing and balance, which are major advantages for survival. Mammals have four different types of hair cell, two of which are dedicated to hearing, the inner and outer hair cells, and the other two to balance, the type-I and type-II hair cells. While all hair cells employ common mechanisms to detect and relay signals from sound or motion, they also have unique attributes that specialise them for a specific functional role. In this chapter we describe the process of signal transmission in mammalian auditory and vestibular hair cells. Since mammalian hair cells do not regenerate, their loss results in permanent auditory or vestibular deficit. Efforts to regenerate or repair malfunctioning hair cells have recently intensified, mainly through gene, stem-cell and molecular therapy.

Keywords: hair cell, cochlea, vestibular, ion channel, ribbon synapse, stem cell, gene therapy

1. Introduction

The inner ear of vertebrates houses the auditory and the vestibular systems. Hearing and balance are key senses that allow humans and other vertebrates to acquire important information from the surrounding environment and to detect and compensate for head motion. The receptors responsible for these sensory functions are the hair cells. The defining feature of hair cells is the presence of the hair bundle that protrudes from their apical surface (**Figure 1A** and **B**). The hair bundle is composed of many microvilli-like structures, termed stereocilia, organised in rows of increasing height. The individual stereocilia are connected to one another by different types of membranous linkages, which ensure that the whole hair bundle moves as one functional unit in response to sensory stimulation. One of these links is the tip-link that connects the tip of each shorter stereocilia to the side of the taller adjacent stereocilia (**Figure 1C**). Tip links are composed of cadherin 23 at the upper end, forming the insertion point on the taller stereocilia, and protocadherin 15 at the lower end that connects to the tip of the shorter stereocilia [2] (**Figure 1D**). The lower end of

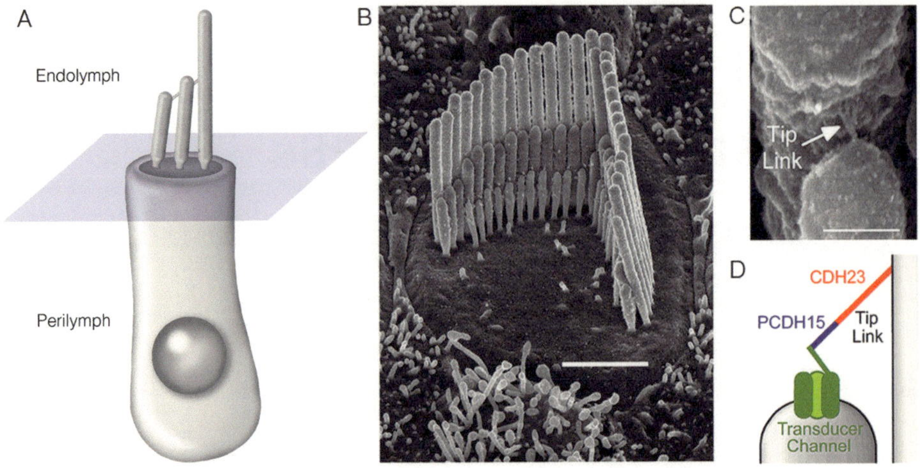

Figure 1.
Hair cell morphology. (A) Cartoon of a generic hair cell. (B) Scanning electron microscope (SEM) image showing the structure of the hair bundle from a cochlear outer hair cell, with the characteristic staircase structure composed of rows of stereocilia of decreasing height. Scale bar: 2 μm. (C) High magnification SEM of a tip link connecting adjacent stereocilia from a cochlear inner hair cell. Scale bar: 200 nm. (D) Drawing showing the tip link connecting the MET channel to the adjacent taller stereocilia. CDH23, cadherin 23; PCDH15, protocadherin 15. Figure modified with permission from Marcotti [1].

the tip-link joins to a protein complex containing the mechanosensitive, non-selective cation-permeable, ion channel, the so called mechanoelectrical transducer (MET) channel (**Figure 1D**). The best candidate for the MET channel pore is the transmembrane channel-like 1 (TMC1) protein, which has ten transmembrane domains [3, 4]. Mutations of TMC1 results in deafness [5]. Notably, persistent TMC2 expression in vestibular hair cells (TMC2 is only expressed during development in cochlear hair cells) may preserve vestibular function in humans with hearing loss caused by TMC1 mutations [6].

The structural polarisation of the stereocilia gives the hair bundle its axis of mechanical sensitivity. When the sensory-evoked motion of fluid around the hair bundle deflects it towards the taller stereocilia, the tension on the tip links increases and the MET channels open [7]. This allows cations to enter the stereocilia and depolarise the hair cell from its resting membrane potential. Depolarization is graded with the amplitude of the MET current since mature hair cells do not fire action potentials. Deflection of the hair bundle in the opposite direction reduces the tension in the tip links and the MET channels close. In the absence of sensory input, the hair bundle is stationary in its resting position. At rest, there is a slight tension on the tip links that opens a proportion of the MET channels resulting in an inward resting transducer current, which depolarises the resting membrane potential of the hair cells and drives a resting discharge of action potentials in the primary sensory neurons [8, 9].

A crucial feature for hair cell function is the tight separation of the fluid surrounding the apical hair bundle from that surrounding the basolateral cell body (**Figure 1A**). In mammals, the hair bundle is bathed in endolymph, a unique extracellular solution, with a high K^+ (157 mM), low Na^+ (1 mM) and very low Ca^{2+} concentration (20–40 μM) [10, 11]. The hair cell body is surrounded by perilymph, a normal extracellular solution with low K^+ (4 mM) and high Na^+ (148 mM) and Ca^{2+} (1.3 mM) concentrations. Potassium is actively secreted into the endolymph by specialised non-sensory epithelial cells found in both the vestibular organs, the vestibular dark cells, and in the *scala media* of the cochlea, the marginal cells of the *stria vascularis* [12]. In the cochlea, this creates a large electrical potential difference of 80–90 mV between the endolymph and perilymph, called the endocochlear potential (EP) [13]; in vestibular organs, the electrical potential difference is much smaller: 1–11 mV ([14] for a recent review see [15]). Since the hair cell resting potential is around −60 mV, there is a large electrical driving force for K^+ entry into the hair cells, via the MET channels, of around 150 mV in the cochlea and 70 mV in the vestibular apparatus. This scenario not only allows a very efficient depolarisation of the hair cells but also provides a route for cell repolarisation since K^+ is able to move out of the cell down a large concentration gradient into the perilymph surrounding its basolateral membrane.

The hair cell receptor potential is shaped by the interplay of the depolarising MET current together with the current through voltage-gated ion channels in the hair cell basolateral membrane (**Figure 2**). Hair cell repolarisation is governed by the exit of K^+ ions through different types of voltage-gated K^+ channel that differ in terms of their kinetics and voltage sensitivity. The depolarising phase of the receptor potential also activates basolateral voltage-gated Ca^{2+} channels that allow Ca^{2+} entry into the hair cell. The influx of Ca^{2+} triggers the release of the neurotransmitter glutamate from specialised ribbon synapses onto postsynaptic afferent fibres (**Figure 2**). Ribbons are electron-dense presynaptic organelles that tether kinetically distinct pools of synaptic vesicles close to the presynaptic membrane [17–19]. The large pools of vesicles allow hair cells to maintain rapid rates of neurotransmitter release and respond to sensory stimulation over prolonged periods of time [18, 20]. Glutamate binds to α-amino-3-hydroxy-5-methyl-4-isoxazolepropionic acid (AMPA)-type glutamate receptors on the postsynaptic afferent fibres [21–23], triggering action potential activity that is relayed to the brain.

The general process of signal transduction and transmission described above is similar for all hair cells, but mammalian auditory and vestibular hair cells have evolved unique mechanisms and attributes, over hundreds of millions of years, that specialise them to perform specific functional roles. There are four types of hair cell in the mammalian inner ear (**Figure 2**): the inner hair cells (IHCs) and outer hair cells (OHCs) in the cochlea, and the type-I and type-II hair cells in the vestibular organs, which include the saccule, the utricle, and the semicircular canals. In the cochlea, the IHCs are the main sensory receptors whose role is to convert acoustic information into electrical activity and relay it to the spiral ganglion neurons (SGNs), the primary sensory neurons. The OHCs, on the other hand, respond to the same stimulation by changing their length, a unique property called electromotility [24]. So rather than being typical sensory hair cells, the cochlear OHCs form the so called "cochlear amplifier" where their main function is to amplify and fine-tune sound-evoked input to the IHCs, increasing hearing sensitivity and frequency discrimination [7].

In contrast to the auditory hair cells, both the type-I and type-II hair cells in the vestibular system have a sensory role. Type-II hair cells are cylindrically shaped and are contacted by several afferent fibres, similar to auditory IHCs (**Figure 2**). Type-I hair cells have a distinguishing flask-shaped appearance, and their basolateral membrane is almost completely enveloped by a single giant calyx-like expansion formed by a single afferent nerve terminal (**Figure 2**). Type-I hair cells are only present in amniotes, and their appearance with evolution has been associated with the transition to life on dry land and rapid head movements [25]. A lot of progress has been made in understanding the intimate functional and molecular mechanisms of hair cell function using a combination of genetics, structural biology, and electrophysiology. In this

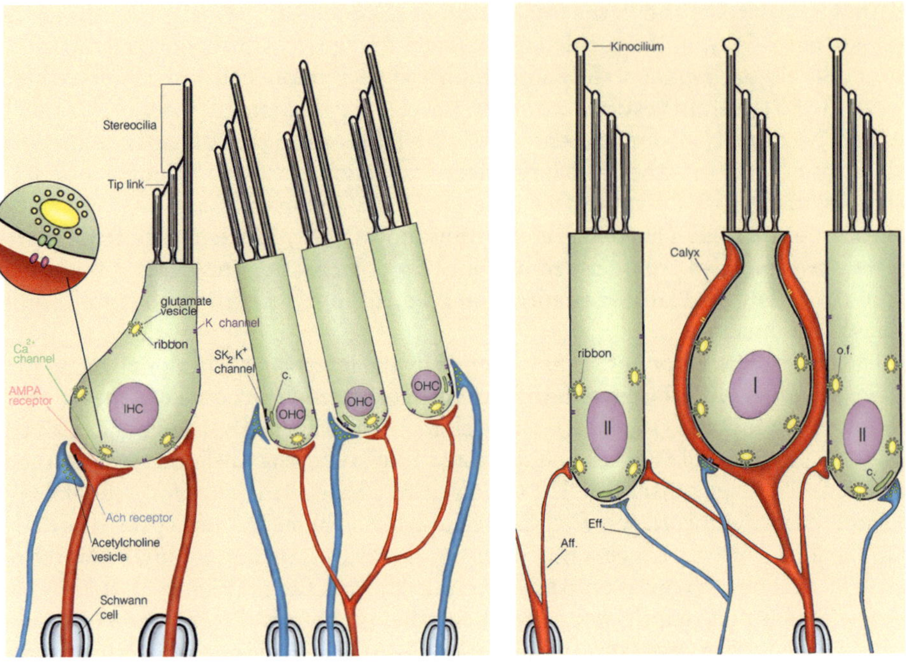

Figure 2.
Auditory and vestibular hair cells and their innervation in adult mammals. Left: in the cochlea, Bouton afferent nerve terminals (red) occur at the basolateral membrane and face a single ellipsoid synaptic body (ribbon, large yellow oval) per active zone in both IHCs and OHCs – Some terminals are not shown in figure for clarity. Presynaptic vesicles (yellow filled circles) containing the afferent neurotransmitter (glutamate) are shown tethered to the ribbon. Voltage-gated $Ca_V1.3$ Ca^{2+} channels (green) are clustered at the presynaptic membrane, opposed to glutamatergic AMPA receptors (magenta) at the afferent postsynaptic membrane. The zoom shows a presynaptic zone facing the postsynaptic membrane. IHCs only form afferent synapses (5 to 30) with type I (myelinated) spiral ganglion neurons (SGNs), which represent ~95% of all SGNs. OHCs form afferent synapses with the remaining ~5% type II (unmyelinated) SGNs. Each type I SGN only forms a single synaptic contact with a single IHC. By contrast, each type II SGN contacts several OHCs. Efferent Bouton nerve terminals (blue) synapse onto type I SGN boutons in close proximity to IHCs (unmyelinated lateral olivocochlear (LOC) neurons), or directly contact OHCs (myelinated medial olivocochlear (MOC) neurons). Only a single LOC efferent is shown for clarity while, in reality, a rich plexus of endings is formed beneath each IHC. Presynaptic vesicles (green filled circles) containing the efferent neurotransmitter (acetylcholine) are also shown. Cholinergic receptors (blue) facing the efferent terminal are located at the OHC postsynaptic membrane, and at the afferent Bouton contacting the IHC. The efferent synapse onto OHCs is marked by a subsynaptic cistern (c.). right: in the vestibular epithelia, afferent nerve terminals (red) are myelinated and are classified as calyx-only if they only contact type-I HCs, dimorphic if they contact both type-I and type-II HCs, and Bouton-only if they only contact type-II HCs. Each Bouton afferent terminal faces a single ribbon, whereas each calyx is opposed to several (7–20) ribbons. Efferent neurons (blue) originating in the brainstem directly contact several type-II HCs and may also contact calyces and boutons. An outer face (o.f.) synapse between the type-II hair cell and the calyx is also shown [16], whose function remains to be elucidated. Note that a single eccentric cilium called kinocilium, which is found adjacent to the longest stereocilia row, is present in mature vestibular hair cells but not in cochlear hair cells which lose it during maturation. The kinocilium is likely involved in the morphogenesis of the hair bundle during embryonic development, while the reason for its persistence in mature vestibular hair cells is unknown.

chapter, we describe the current understanding of signal processing and transmission by the different mammalian hair cell types.

The differentiation of auditory or vestibular hair cells from common cell precursors is guided by an extensive array of molecules, expressed with a highly ordered spatiotemporal pattern, which is only recently beginning to be understood [26–29]. The cost of such an elaborate program of differentiation is that the mammalian inner ear is unable to replace hair cells loss due to, for example, damage, genetic mutation or ageing. More and more gene mutations are becoming identified that produce, or cause predisposition to, inner ear disorders due to hair cell malfunction or even death [30, 31]. At the end of this chapter, we look at the different strategies that are being developed as potential therapies to regenerate hair cells or to restore their function.

2. The inner ear

2.1 Signal processing in the cochlea

The mammalian auditory system can sense and transmit different acoustic features such as sound frequency, intensity, timing and duration, all of which have vast dynamic ranges. Humans, for example, have a hearing frequency range spanning three orders of magnitude, from 20 Hz to 20 kHz or approximately 10 octaves, and can detect sound intensity differences of over 12 orders of magnitude, up to 120 dB. We can discriminate small sound level differences with nearly constant acuity (~1 dB) across almost the entire range [32, 33]. In order to achieve this, the mammalian cochlea has evolved a number of different strategies. The cochlea has a spiralled structure and contains around 3500 IHCs and three times as many OHCs. Sound enters the cochlea via the ear drum and the ossicles in the middle ear. The cochlea is tonotopically organised, such that hair cells at the base of the spiral respond best to high-frequency sound, and cells at the apex respond best to the lowest frequencies. Cochlear tonotopy is primarily imposed by the mechanical properties of the basilar membrane upon which the hair cells reside, which is wider and more flexible at the apical low frequency end and narrower and stiffer at the basal high frequency end [34]. Sound causes a wave that travels along the basilar membrane with the largest oscillation occurring at the base of the cochlea for high frequency sounds and towards the apex for lower frequencies [13]. The movement produced by the oscillation of the basilar membrane causes the hair bundles of the IHCs and OHCs to move back and forth at the sound frequency, opening and closing the MET channels, creating a receptor potential in the hair cells. The sinusoidal change in receptor potential modulates neurotransmitter exocytosis in IHCs and electromotility in the OHCs [35, 36]. The combined electromotile activity of the three rows of OHCs amplifies the sound-induced motion of the basilar membrane. Cochlear amplification ensures that each IHC is sharply tuned to a narrow sound frequency band, known as its *characteristic frequency* (CF) (for a review see [37]).

The tonotopic organisation of the cochlea translates the frequency code of sound into a place code. Each IHC along the cochlea represents a narrowly tuned frequency channel, like the keys on a piano, that form a tonotopic frequency map. This map is preserved and represented throughout the auditory pathway, all the way to the cortex. A sound frequency is therefore represented by the relative position of the active IHC, or neurons, within the tonotopic map, rather than being encoded by the receptor potential or neuronal firing rates; although this does also occur for frequencies below a few KHz (see next section). While sound frequency is represented by the tonotopic map and split among all the IHCs within each cochlea, the duration, timing and entire intensity range has to be encoded by neurotransmitter release from every IHC and distributed among the afferent nerve fibres of SGNs, which are estimated to be about 35,000–50,000 [38]. The functional mechanisms underlying IHC sound processing are described in the following section.

2.1.1 Cochlear inner hair cells

The IHCs convert the sound-induced motion of the hair bundle into a receptor potential that drives neurotransmitter release onto auditory afferent neurons. For frequencies below ~2 kHz, the IHC receptor potential follows the MET current with cycles of depolarisation and hyperpolarisation at the stimulating sound frequency. Therefore, the receptor potential of low frequency IHCs is dominated by an alternating current 'AC' component that 'phase-locks' to the sound frequency [39, 40]. The magnitude of the AC component is proportional to the size of the MET current, which is greater for louder sounds [39, 41]. Above a few kilohertz, the filtering properties of the IHC membrane prevents the receptor potential from phase-locking. As such, high frequency IHCs respond to sound with a depolarising shift in membrane potential, a direct current 'DC' component, that is sustained for the duration of the sound. As for the AC component, the magnitude of the DC component is proportional to the loudness [41, 42].

The receptor potentials of low- and high-frequency IHCs are determined by the interaction of the MET current with that through different voltage-dependent Ca^{2+} and K^+ channels expressed in their basolateral membrane. About 90% of the Ca^{2+} current in all IHCs is carried by $Ca_V1.3$ Ca^{2+} channels [43, 44]. Consistent with a crucial role of $Ca_V1.3$ Ca^{2+} channels in IHC signal transmission, deletion of $Ca_V1.3$ in mice [44, 45] or loss of its function in humans [46] produces deafness. The Ca^{2+} channels provide the inward Ca^{2+} current that is vital for IHC depolarization as well as for triggering exocytosis (see below). Adult mouse IHCs also have several different K^+ channel types that provide the outward K^+ current required for cell repolarisation and for setting the resting membrane potential. There is a voltage-dependent K^+ current characterised by slow activation kinetics (I_{Ks}), a negatively activating delayed-rectifier K^+ current ($I_{K,n}$), and a large voltage- and Ca^{2+}-dependent K^+ current characterised by fast activation kinetics (I_{Kf}) [47–49]. Several K^+ channel subunits have been identified so far, which account for the above K^+ currents: Kv1.8, Kv7.4, Kv11.1, and Kv12.1 for I_{Ks}, $KCNQ_4$ (Kv7.4) for $I_{K,n}$, and BK_{Ca} channels for I_{Kf} [50]. Consistent with the different receptor potential responses of low- and high-frequency cells, tonotopic differences in the biophysical characteristics of IHCs combine to optimise IHC responses to acoustic stimuli of different frequency [51]. Low frequency IHCs have a large MET channel resting open probability (>40% open at rest in physiological conditions) compared to that in high frequency cells (<10%), resulting in the former having a more depolarised resting potential [51]. Low frequency IHCs also have a different complement of voltage-gated K^+ channels compared to high-frequency cells [51]. For low frequency IHCs, the depolarised resting potential activates a large proportion of the basolateral membrane currents, to increase the speed and accuracy of the frequency-following component of the receptor potential [50, 51]. For high frequency IHCs, the more hyperpolarised resting potential and smaller proportion of currents active at rest allow the responses of these cells to summate into a DC membrane potential shift proportional to stimulus intensity [51]. Therefore, both low and high frequency IHCs are intrinsically tuned to accurately represent the main component of the cells' *in vivo* receptor potential, showing a preference for either timing (AC) or intensity (DC) coding, respectively. While low frequency IHCs respond rapidly and accurately to phasic stimuli up to the phase-locking limit, high frequency cells respond with clearly defined graded shifts in membrane potential over an extended dynamic range.

The specialisation of low and high frequency IHCs for either response timing or graded accuracy, respectively, is likely to be related to the main mechanisms used for localising low or high frequency sounds. In mammals, low frequencies are localised using the inter-aural timing difference (ITD) of a sound arriving at the two ears, by the CNS comparing the differences in timing of the phase-locked activity in auditory afferents [52]. High frequency sounds are conversely localised using the inter-aural level difference (ILD) of a sound between the two ears, by comparing differences in the level of activity in the afferents [53]. Therefore, the IHC biophysical properties are best suited to maximise the accuracy of response-timing in low frequency cells and response-level in high frequency cells, allowing the detection of ITDs as small as 10 ms and ILDs of only 1–2 dB [54]. As well as the differences in their biophysical properties, IHCs also show tonotopic differences in the number, organisation and function of their ribbon synapses that favour transmission of the intrinsic tuning for either phasic or graded receptor potentials (see below).

All of the acoustic information encoded in the IHC receptor potential, including timing, intensity and duration, has to be faithfully encoded by neurotransmitter release at the IHC ribbon synapses into activity in the SGNs. Each IHC has between 5 and 30 presynaptic active zones [55] with a specialised synaptic ribbon and post-synaptic afferent bouton from an unbranched type-I SGN [56, 57] (**Figure 2**). The individual ribbon synapses within each IHC have different activation ranges, presumably to extend the range of stimulus intensities transmitted by each IHC [58–61]. As well as differences between individual synapses there are also tonotopic differences in the overall synaptic function of IHCs, which could represent a sound frequency-dependent tuning of exocytosis that correlates with the specialisation for phasic or graded receptor potentials described above. In the following paragraphs we will focus on these tonotopic specialisations and how they relate to the different receptor characteristics of low and high frequency IHCs.

The IHC synaptic ribbons are electron-dense presynaptic organelles, composed mainly of the protein ribeye [62]. The function of the synaptic ribbon is to tether kinetically distinct pools of synaptic vesicles close to the release sites to provide a rapid and relatively inexhaustible release of the neurotransmitter glutamate in response to acoustic stimulation (for recent reviews see [19, 63, 64]). The vesicles attached to the base of the ribbon and docked at the presynaptic active zones form the readily releasable pool (RRP), consisting of a few hundred vesicles per IHC [17–19], and are the first to be released following stimulation. The ribbon associated vesicles that are further away from the release sites together form a larger secondarily releasable pool (SRP), which is believed to refill the RRP once it has become depleted to maintain relatively high rates of exocytosis for long periods of stimulation [19, 63, 64].

As mentioned above, exocytosis of glutamate-containing synaptic vesicles at IHC ribbon synapses is triggered by the entry of Ca^{2+} through closely coupled voltage-gated $Ca_V1.3$ Ca^{2+}channels in response to cell depolarisation, similar to conventional synapses. These channels are suited for driving neurotransmitter release at sensory synapses since they activate at around, or below, the IHCs estimated resting potential (about −60 mV: [51, 65, 66]). $Ca_V1.3$ channels also show rapid activation kinetics (sub-millisecond), which is required for precise timing [65–67], and little voltage- or Ca^{2+}-dependent inactivation, allowing them to drive prolonged or continuous neurotransmission [45, 68]. Unlike conventional synapses, however, many of the established synaptic proteins have not been found at ribbon synapses, such as the SNARE proteins [69] nor the traditional Ca^{2+} sensors of exocytosis, synaptotagmin

1 and 2 [64, 70]. Instead, IHC ribbon synapses are likely to rely on the function of the ribbon itself, along with the structural proteins bassoon and piccolino (for reviews see [19, 63, 64]) and the multifunctional role of the Ca^{2+} binding protein otoferlin [71–73]. Otoferlin has multiple Ca^{2+} binding domains and is considered to be the main Ca^{2+} sensor for synaptic vesicle exocytosis at IHCs ribbon synapses with multiple roles in the synaptic vesicle cycle, including vesicle priming, docking, fusion, vesicle pool replenishment and endocytosis [19, 20, 71, 72]. Consistent with the primary role of otoferlin in IHCs, *otoferlin* knockout mice are deaf, and mutations in human otoferlin causes a nonsyndromic form of deafness [71, 74].

As well as otoferlin, the Ca^{2+} dependence of neurotransmitter release at IHC ribbon synapses has been shown to be dependent on the unconventional synaptotagmin isoform, synaptotagmin 4 (Syt4) [75]. Synaptotagmin 4 is unusual since it does not bind Ca^{2+} in the normal Ca^{2+} sensing domain for exocytosis [76] and, as such, is believed to work together with otoferlin to decrease the overall Ca^{2+} dependence of exocytosis in mature IHCs [75]. The Ca^{2+} dependence of IHC synaptic vesicle release determines its operating range and sensitivity to both small and large fluctuations in the cell receptor potential. This important property has been studied in IHCs from different cochlear regions using patch clamp to record Ca^{2+} currents and changes in cell membrane capacitance (ΔC_m) that are indicative of exocytosis from the cells complement of ribbon synapses [75, 77–82]. In mature IHCs, neurotransmitter release is graded with cell membrane depolarization and, apart from very low-frequency IHCs (see below), is linearly dependent on Ca^{2+} entry [78, 79, 83]. Such a linear relation seems to be a feature of many sensory synapses where graded amounts of neurotransmitter release are required [19]. The functional significance of the linear relation is likely to be that it extends the dynamic range of sound intensity discrimination by facilitating exocytosis at low levels, as well as preventing synapse saturation at high levels. While this is true for high frequency IHCs, such as those in the mouse (sensitive to sounds above a few kHz), very low frequency cells, such as those of the gerbil (CF around 300 Hz) have a high-order exocytotic Ca^{2+} dependence [80, 81]. Such supralinear relation is thought to emphasise the phasic component of the receptor potential to accurately localise very low frequency sounds [51, 81].

While the mechanism responsible for the tonotopic differences in IHC Ca^{2+} dependence remains unknown, the linear relation seems to be correlated with the presence of Syt4, with high frequency mouse and gerbil IHCs showing its expression whereas it is absent from low frequency gerbil IHCs [75]. This suggests that the Ca^{2+} dependence could be determined by the intrinsic properties of the Ca^{2+} sensor, which is likely to be otoferlin, with or without Syt4. Alternatively, such differences could also arise from a variation in the topographic coupling of Ca^{2+} channels and vesicle release sites [55, 78]. It has been suggested that a linear exocytotic Ca^{2+} dependence could arise from a very close 'nanodomain' coupling between the Ca^{2+} channels and vesicle release sites [78, 84], whereby the opening of a Ca^{2+} channel within a few tens of nanometres from a vesicle, provides enough Ca^{2+} to saturate the Ca^{2+} sensor and trigger vesicle fusion [66, 78]. In this situation, an apparently linear overall relation is created by the one-to-one association of Ca^{2+} channel openings and vesicle release, even though the exocytotic Ca^{2+} sensor has an intrinsically high-order Ca^{2+} dependence [77, 84]. Direct evidence for the nanodomain coupling between Ca^{2+} channels and vesicle release sites in mouse IHCs has come from the finding that the rapidly binding Ca^{2+} chelator BAPTA inhibited exocytosis more than the slowly acting EGTA [82]. However, recent experiments using EGTA showed that exocytosis could be uncoupled from Ca^{2+} entry in high frequency IHCs (CF > 2 kHz) but was more resistant in low frequency cells (CF < 2 kHz) [81]. This implies that high frequency IHCs have a looser 'microdomain'-like coupling whereas low frequency cells have the tighter 'nanodomain' organisation. Therefore, it is likely that the Ca^{2+} dependence of exocytosis is determined by the intrinsic Ca^{2+} binding properties of the Ca^{2+} sensors, as well as the architecture of the ribbon synapses.

The tonotopic differences in the functional characteristics of the IHC synaptic machinery are likely to represent further frequency-specific tuning of the cells to accurately represent the main components of their receptor potential, and optimise the responses of the primary auditory neurons. The high-order exocytotic Ca^{2+} dependence and tight nanodomain coupling of low frequency IHCs, together with their more rapid receptor potential responses (see above), could facilitate the signalling of phase-locked activity up to the highest frequencies possible [51, 81, 85]. By contrast, high frequency IHCs do not follow the frequency component of sound, but instead have to precisely reflect the graded changes in the amplitude and kinetic properties of the macroscopic Ca^{2+} current over a wide dynamic range of sound intensity, which is more in line with a linear Ca^{2+} exocytotic dependence and microdomain coupling involving more than one Ca^{2+} channel [85]. The microdomain coupling of exocytosis is known to enhance the "signal-to-noise" ratio of transmission, by reducing the noise associated with the stochastic Ca^{2+} channel openings [86]. Therefore, mature IHC synapses seem to have developed remarkable frequency-dependent tuning. On one hand low frequency cells show submillisecond encoding of receptor potential fluctuations for accurate phase-locking, while on the other hand, high frequency cells show precise signalling of graded receptor potentials.

A nanodomain coupling of Ca^{2+} channels and synaptic release sites in IHCs that show phase-locked activity to low frequency stimulation has also been suggested from recordings of postsynaptic activity from individual afferent fibres or bouton terminals. The close nanodomain coupling has been used to explain how postsynaptic activity is phase-locked to a particular time point (phase) of the sinusoidal stimulus, independent of its magnitude or intensity [87–90]. In a nanodomain scenario, exocytosis is governed by the properties of the single closely coupled Ca^{2+} channel, such that the increasing channel open probability with depolarization (sound intensity) would similarly increase the fusion probability of the "competent" (nearby) vesicle, resulting in an action potential at the afferent fibre [85]. This scenario could explain why the frequency, but not the amplitude, of EPSCs increases with IHC depolarization [22, 91–93].

It is possible that heterogeneity between individual synapses within the same IHC, in terms of exocytotic Ca^{2+} sensitivity [94], or the size and voltage-dependence of the Ca^{2+} influx [55], could influence the tonotopic variation in the cell's synaptic characteristics. However, differences in the properties of neurotransmitter release among individual synapses, as a function of their tonotopic position along the cochlea, remains unknown. Tonotopic differences have been observed in the spontaneous firing rate of afferent fibres in the gerbil that generally have a higher frequency at the apex than those at base [95], which is likely to reflect the underlying synaptic ribbon function.

2.1.2 Cochlear outer hair cells

Cochlear amplification results from OHC electromotility, whereby the cells change length in response to fluctuations in their receptor potential [37]. For cochlear amplification to work, the motion of the OHCs must follow the stimulating sound on a cycle-by-cycle basis. Therefore, to drive electromotility throughout the entire auditory range, the OHC receptor potential must have an AC component able to accurately follow the MET current up to the highest audible sound frequencies.

The OHCs have, therefore, evolved biophysical specialisations that enhance response speed, which are similar to those described for low-frequency IHCs (see above) and are required to facilitate accurate phase-locking up to a few kHz. The resting open probability of the MET channels in OHCs is about 50% throughout the length of the cochlea when experiments are performed using endolymphatic-like Ca^{2+}concentration [96]. This means that displacement of the stereocilia by the acoustic vibration results in a symmetric sinusoidal voltage excursion of the OHC receptor potential around its resting level. The large resting MET current also means that OHCs have a depolarised resting membrane potential of around −40 mV *in vivo*, which would activate a substantial proportion of the cell's voltage-gated channels.

The predominant voltage-gated K^+ channel expressed in OHCs is $KCNQ_4$ (Kv7.4; [97]) with mutations in $KCNQ_4$ producing deafness [98]. $KCNQ_4$ channels carry the large delayed rectifier K^+ current $I_{K,n}$, defined by its very negative voltage activation range [99]. There is a tonotopic gradient in the size of $I_{K,n}$ with high frequency OHCs having a larger current than that present in low frequency cells [96, 100]. The depolarised resting potential of OHCs would activate over half of the $KCNQ_4$ channels, resulting in high-frequency cells having a larger resting K^+ current (and smaller membrane resistance) than low-frequency cells. There is also a tonotopic difference in the overall size of the OHCs, such that high frequency cells are smaller with lower cell membrane capacitance compared to low frequency cells [43, 96, 100]. Since the cell membrane time constant is determined by the product of cell membrane resistance and membrane capacitance, the smaller values for both in high frequency OHCs greatly increase the speed at which the cells can respond. In fact, the time constant of the OHC membrane was found to be appropriate for allowing voltage responses at their CF as a function of position along the cochlea's tonotopic axis [96]. Therefore, OHCs show frequency-dependent differences in their biophysical properties that tune their voltage responses to CF, with high frequency cells being faster than low frequency cells. The tuning of OHCs is opposite to that seen for IHCs, where very low frequency cells showed the most rapid responses in order to phase-lock to sound up to only a few kHz.

The OHCs also contain $Ca_V1.3$ voltage-gated Ca^{2+} channels [101, 102] that drive the exocytosis of glutamate from their ribbon synapses onto the type-II afferent fibres innervating them. The size of the Ca^{2+} current (measured as a barium current in some studies) in immature and mature OHCs is much smaller than that present in IHCs of comparative ages [75, 102–104], consistent with the presence of fewer synaptic ribbons and afferent terminals on these cells [105]. The voltage dependence of the Ca^{2+} current in mature OHCs was found to be shifted by around 10 mV in the depolarised direction compared to that in IHCs [103], which would have implications on the activity of the Type-II SGNs (discussed below).

The OHC receptor potential is converted into electromotility by the motor protein prestin [106]. The OHCs are unique in that they are the only cells known to be endowed with somatic electromotility. Prestin is encoded by the *SLC26A5* gene, a member of the SLC26 anion transporter family [106] which has, however, lost its transport function [107]. Prestin is packed in the OHC lateral membrane at an amazingly high density of over 10,000/μm^2 [108]. In response to the sinusoidal depolarization produced by the MET current during acoustic stimulation, prestin acts as a reverse piezoelectric, by mechanically changing its conformation as a function of voltage (see [37]). As a result, OHC depolarization or hyperpolarisation shortens or lengthens the OHC, respectively, by a few μm. Since the tips of the OHC stereocilia are firmly attached to the underside of the tectorial membrane, unlike those of IHCs, the change in OHC length amplifies the sound-induced oscillation of the local cochlear partition, including the basilar membrane. The result is a stronger mechanical stimulus to the adjacent IHCs, which increases their sensitivity (by as much as 40–60 dB in mice; [109]) and sharpness of frequency tuning. The importance of prestin is also underlined by the finding that mutations produce deafness in humans [110].

Consistent with the local amplifying role of OHCs, they are only contacted by around 5% of all the SGNs in the cochlea, the Type II afferents, which are characterised by thin, unmyelinated axons (**Figure 2**). Each Type II afferent extends hundreds of mm along the cochlear duct to contact several OHCs (up to around 30; [111]). Each OHC, in turn, contacts two to three afferent fibres of Type II SGNs [112]. Exocytosis in OHCs occurs at ribbon synapses, like those of IHCs, with each mature OHC containing only very few ribbons (around 1–4 ribbons per cell: [105]). The presynaptic function of OHCs has been investigated with capacitance measurements only in immature cells andΔ C_m has been found to be much smaller than that of IHCs [75], consistent with their fewer synaptic ribbons. Postsynaptic recordings have shown that, unlike the Type I fibres that contact the IHCs, Type II afferent fibres seem to be activated only when all their OHC inputs are active simultaneously [113, 114]. Such a situation would only by be caused by sounds loud enough to cause acoustic trauma [113, 115, 116], and as such the function of Type II fibres is likely to be related to sensing damage or nociception in the cochlea. Recently, however, it has been shown that Type-II afferents can be activated by non-damaging, loud sounds [117]. The more depolarised activation threshold for the Ca^{2+} current in mature OHCs [103], could be compensated by the much more depolarised *in vivo* resting potential of the OHCs to increase the probability that synapses are simultaneously active. These findings point to a more active role for Type II afferents in auditory signal processing.

Type II activation could be involved in transmitting information to the CNS to activate feedback efferent pathways to reduce cochlear amplification and avoid/limit further damage to the cochlea. The efferent input to the OHC constitutes the majority of their innervation (**Figure 2**). The efferent fibres originate from the medial olivocochlear (MOC) nucleus in the auditory brainstem [118]. Efferent fibres release the neurotransmitter acetylcholine (ACh), the role of which is to inhibit OHC electromotility and hence reduce the mechanical amplification of the cochlear partition [119]. OHC inhibition is achieved because ACh, by promoting Ca^{2+} influx through $\alpha9\alpha10$ nicotinic acetylcholine receptors [120, 121], leads to the opening of co-localised small conductance Ca^{2+}-activated K^+ channels (SK_2: [122]). The efflux of K^+ results in OHC hyperpolarisation. Intracellular Ca^{2+} diffusion away from SK_2 channels is limited by a thin near-membrane cistern that is co-extensive with the efferent terminal contact (**Figure 2**).

2.2 Signal processing in the vestibular organs

In mammals there are five vestibular sensory organs: the two otolith organs, comprising the perpendicularly-arranged utricle and sacculus, and three orthogonally-arranged semicircular canals (horizontal or lateral, anterior, and posterior). The utricle and saccule detect horizontal and vertical linear acceleration, respectively, and contain a sensory epithelium called the *macula*, composed of a flat sheet of sensory hair cells and supporting cells. The hair cell stereocilia project into the gelatinous otolithic membrane that has otoliths, or ear stones, on its upper surface. The semicircular canals detect angular acceleration in the three spatial dimensions and contain a sensory epithelium that is called the *crista,* which is similar to the *macula* but smaller. In the *crista* the hair cell hair bundles project into the gelatinous cupula. On average, there are around 10,000 vestibular hair cells in each mouse labyrinth, distributed nearly equally between otolith and canal epithelia [123]. As mentioned in the introduction, vestibular hair cells are subdivided into type-I and type-II cells based on their cell body shape and innervation pattern [16, 123–127] (see **Figure 2**). The sensory epithelia in the vestibular organs act as accelerometers, detecting motion due to linear or angular acceleration and gravity. These forces act on the otolithic membrane or the cupula and, combined with the inertia of the endolymph within the vestibular organs, deflects the hair bundles of both type-I and type-II hair cells. This activates vestibular hair cell signal transduction and information is relayed to the brain via the vestibular afferent fibres. Vestibular information is used centrally to drive several motor reflexes. These include the incredibly fast vestibulo-ocular reflex that maintains eye position and gaze stabilisation [128], and those controlling balance and posture [129]. Vestibular information is also used to generate spatial memory, and to support orientation and navigation of an individual in the environment [130, 131]. When vestibular signalling is impaired, disabling pathological conditions arise such as vertigo, nausea, ataxia, an altered perception of self-orientation and oscillopsia.

The vestibular system is considered to be a low-frequency analyser since it provides information about velocity of naturally occurring head movements at frequencies ranging from 0.1 to a few tens of Hz, well below the frequency of acoustic stimuli sensed by cochlear hair cells [132, 133]. Therefore, there is no graded organisation of the hair cells according to their characteristic frequency, as observed in the cochlea [51]. In the vestibular sensory epithelia, hair cells are instead arranged in two different zones. In the *maculae* of the otolithic organs, there is a curved central stripe, called the striola, that shows distinct morpho-functional properties with respect to the remaining outer area of the sensory epithelium, called the extrastriolar region. There is a similar distinction in the *cristae*, with a central zone being equivalent in many ways to the striolar region of the macula, and a peripheral zone that is similar to the extrastriolar region (reviewed in [25]). One major functional difference between the zones relates to the firing activity in the afferent fibres that contact the hair cells. In the striolar and central zones, afferents show highly irregular spike activity and adapting responses to head motion, which are best suited for encoding rapid phasic signals (transient motions; [123]). By contrast, afferents from the extrastriolar and peripheral zones show regular tonic spike trains, suitable for encoding slow movements and sustained stimuli, such as maintained head tilts and gravity [123, 124, 134, 135].

The correlation between hair cell type and the zonal segregation is less clear, since both type-I and type-II hair cells are distributed throughout the vestibular sensory epithelia. There is, however, a zonal difference in the afferent wiring patterns of the hair cells. Hair cells transmit their signal onto three different classes of vestibular afferents. The calyx-only afferents only innervate type-I hair cells, with the calyx almost completely enclosing the basolateral surface of the hair cell, and can surround a single, or multiple, type-I cells. Bouton-only afferents have smaller terminals, similar to those on cochlear hair cells, and branch to innervate several type-II hair cells. Finally, dimorphic afferents represent the majority of vestibular afferents and are branched to form both calyx endings on type-I hair cells and bouton terminals on type-II hair cells [132, 135, 136] (**Figure 2**). While both calyceal and bouton terminals are found throughout the vestibular sensory epithelium, afferents in central/striolar zones are either calyx-only or dimorphic, such that all irregularly firing afferents receive a proportion of their input from type-I hair cells. Afferents in peripheral/extrastriolar zones are either bouton-only or dimorphic, such that all regularly firing afferents contact at least one type-II hair cell. Therefore, while there is a degree of overlap from the dimorphic afferents, it grossly appears that type-I hair cells are responsible for the rapid phasic component of the afferent response, while type-II hair cells are required for the tonic component.

2.2.1 Vestibular type-I and type-II hair cells

Both type-I and type-II hair cells transduce head motion into a firing activity within the vestibular ganglion neurons. A major goal of vestibular neuroscience is to understand the distinct functional roles of type-I and type-II hair cells. It is thought that type-I hair cells and their encapsulating calyces might have evolved more recently in amniotes (anamniotes only have type-II hair cells) to allow more rapid transmission of information, possibly required for the transition to a land-based life and the acquisition of a head moving independently of the body trunk [25].

The receptor potential in both type-I and type-II vestibular hair cells is driven by the depolarizing current flowing through MET channels following sensory-evoked displacement of the hair bundles [137, 138], as for cochlear hair cells. Hair cell depolarisation then activates voltage-gated K^+ channels expressed in their basolateral membrane, the opening of which results in cell repolarisation [139, 140]. While this mechanism is similar to that of cochlear hair cells, the complement of underlying K^+ channels differs not only with cochlear hair cells but also between type-I and type-II hair cells. In type-II hair cells, the total outward K^+ current is composed of a delayed-rectifying current, an A-type inactivating current, and a Ca^{2+}-activated K^+ current. Type-II hair cells also express the hyperpolarisation-activated (anomalous rectifying) K^+ current and the mixed Na^+/K^+ permeable I_h [141]. As well as an I_h current [141], type-I hair cells have a delayed rectifier K^+ current component, together with a large outwardly rectifying K^+ current, termed $I_{K,L}$, that activates at very hyperpolarised membrane potentials, such that it is about half activated at the hair cell's resting membrane potential of around −70 mV ([142–144]; see [28] for a comparison of ion channels expressed in auditory and vestibular sensory epithelia). The molecular identity of the channel carrying $I_{K,L}$ remains unknown, however, both KCNQ and ether-a-go-go (erg) K^+ channel subunits have been suggested to contribute [145]. The substantial activation of $I_{K,L}$ at the resting potential of type-I hair cells means that these cells have a significantly lower resting membrane resistance (typically less than 50 MΩ) compared to type-II hair cells (about 1 GΩ) [142, 143, 146]. Since the speed of the cells' voltage responses is determined by the membrane time constant, the low membrane resistance of type-I hair cells means they have faster but smaller voltage responses compared to type-II hair cells (see [147]). This is consistent with the different functional roles proposed for type-I and type-II hair cells as either rapid phasic receptors or slower graded receptors, respectively.

The transmission of vestibular information from the hair cells takes place at the interface between the cells and the afferent terminals. As for auditory hair cells, this occurs at ribbon synapses present in both types of vestibular hair cell, where the Ca^{2+}-dependent release of glutamate triggers an action potential discharge at the postsynaptic terminals [16, 21, 23, 126, 137]. An important difference is that while each auditory afferent receives the sensory input from a single ribbon, multiple ribbons contribute the sensory input to a single vestibular afferent due to their branching (**Figure 2**). Therefore, each vestibular neuron integrates the information from several type-I and/or type-II hair cells. In the case of the calyx, there is an additional integration of information from the multiple ribbon synapses in each type-I hair cell it surrounds. As well as the quantal release of glutamate, type-I hair cells have been shown to use a non-quantal mechanism of signal transmission that relies on the unique architecture of the postsynaptic calyx [25, 148, 149]. The two modes of vestibular hair cell transmission are described below.

The process of quantal synaptic transmission in both vestibular hair cell types is similar to that described above for IHCs. Both type-I and type-II hair cells have similar numbers of synaptic ribbons, ranging from 7 to 20 per cell [21, 23, 126]. The fusion of synaptic vesicles at the ribbon synapse release sites is triggered by Ca^{2+} influx through $Ca_V1.3$ Ca^{2+} channels, and mediated by the Ca^{2+} sensor of exocytosis otoferlin [21, 23, 139, 150–153]. Mature utricular type-II hair cells have a relatively large RRP and SRP of synaptic vesicles that become recruited following sustained stimulation [153–155]. The large synaptic vesicle pools in type-II cells, which are similar in size to those in mature IHCs, allow them to sustain the transmission of tonic signals. This is important for maintaining head orientation relative to gravity and for encoding slowly varying signals such as low-frequency head movements during walking or running [156]. Mature utricular type-I hair cells, on the other hand, show much less synaptic vesicle exocytosis, with an RRP, which is around an order of magnitude smaller than that in type-II hair cells, and little evidence of an SRP [153]. Although the overall amount of exocytosis differs between type-I and type-II hair cells, the number of vesicles released in the RRP of a mature type-I cell onto a single calyx is likely to be comparable to the amount of RRP vesicles released by type-II cells onto a single afferent terminal [153]. The relatively small degree of exocytosis in mature type-I hair cells is likely to be a developmental adaptation since it is much larger at immature stages [21, 72].

In mature utricular type-II hair cells neurotransmitter release has a high-order Ca^{2+} dependence [153–155], similar to that found in low frequency mature IHCs [81]. The Ca^{2+} dependence of the smaller exocytotic component in mature type-I hair cells remains to be established. A high-order relation in vestibular hair cells could be beneficial for representing phasic receptor potentials with speed and fidelity [51, 81]. Differences in the properties of exocytosis between vestibular hair cells located in different regions of the vestibular organs (*e.g.*, striola/central compared to extrastriola/peripheral), remains to be determined.

While postsynaptic recordings have been made from the calyces of type-I hair cells [21, 23], no such data is available from the bouton terminals on type-II cells. However, a comparison of EPSCs recorded from vestibular calyces and the boutons innervating mature cochlear IHCs [92] reveals differences that reflect the presynaptic findings described above. The overall size of individual EPSCs is much smaller in calyces compared to IHC boutons, and there is an increase in EPSC amplitude with type-I hair cell depolarization that is not seen at cochlear boutons. Calyceal EPSCs have an unusually wide range of decays time constants, with some being very slow, presumably reflecting a substantial glutamate accumulation and spill over in the calyceal synaptic cleft [23]. The accumulation and spill over of glutamate within the very restricted volume of the synaptic cleft would provide a high synaptic gain to maximise the effect of the relatively small amount of glutamate release on the calyceal terminal. A more restricted release of glutamate from type-I hair cells could also prevent glutamate from rising to cytotoxic levels within the synaptic cleft during prolonged stimulation.

This could be a reason why a large, and potentially damaging, SRP in type-I hair cells may have been replaced by an alternative non-quantal mechanism of signal transmission [25].

Evidence for a non-quantal mode of transmission in type-I hair cells comes from the fact that neither *Ca*$_V$*1.3* nor *otoferlin* knockout mouse models show any serious vestibular deficit [71, 157]. Moreover, robust action potential activity could be elicited by hair cell depolarization in calyces from mature *Ca*$_V$*1.3* or *otoferlin* knockout mice, which was not affected by the AMPA receptor antagonist NBQX [153]. It is, therefore, possible that the lack of glutamate exocytosis in these transgenic mice is compensated by non-quantal, Ca^{2+} independent signal transmission which has been shown to occur between type-I hair cells and their surrounding calyx terminal ([137, 158–161]; recently reviewed in [148, 149]). However, the capacity of non-quantal transmission to sustain vestibular function in the absence of chemical neurotransmission, requires further detailed investigation.

While the exact mechanism of non-quantal transmission remains unknown, it appears to involve voltage-gated K^+ channels expressed in the pre- and post-synaptic membranes facing the synaptic cleft [146, 162]. Different modes of action have been hypothesised, although they are not mutually exclusive: 1) K^+ exit from the basolateral membrane of the type-I hair cells directly depolarizes the calyx by changing the Nernst equilibrium potential across the inner calyx membrane [146, 155, 158, 159, 162]; 2) pre- and post-synaptic K^+ channels create a resistive coupling which allows for a direct (electrical) depolarization of the calyx [159] – note that electrical transmission typically involves gap junctions that are not present in the type-I hair cell-calyx synapse [125, 137]; 3) an ephaptic mechanism, whereby electrical fields created across narrowing and invagination of the synaptic space [125], can near-instantaneously influence the electrical excitability of the calyx [163], although there is currently no experimental support for this hypothesis.

The reasons why type-I vestibular hair cells require a dual, quantal and non-quantal, mode of signal transmission, are not clear. A restricted RRP of synaptic vesicles [153] might provide a transient (phasic) pulse of depolarization to the calyx, presumably to emphasise the transient component of the stimulus, as observed in calyceal afferents [123]. The potentially slower but sustained non-quantal transmission due to the accumulation of K^+ or glutamate in the synaptic cleft following hair cell depolarisation [23, 146] would provide a graded and tonic component of transmission or a sustained baseline level of calyx stimulation, which amplifies the effect of quantal transmission. Alternatively or additionally, if non-quantal transmission is a resistive or ephaptic coupling, it would provide a very fast (sub-millisecond) signal component [25, 137, 159, 164]. Such rapid transmission might be required for signalling jerk (the onset of acceleration: [164]) and for driving the rapid vestibulo-ocular reflex (VOR). The VOR, which stabilises gaze by counter-rotating the eyes during head rotation, is the fastest known reflex with a total latency as small as ~5 ms in the rhesus monkey [165].

While the exact functional roles of type-I and type-II vestibular hair cells remain to be determined, their very different biophysics and mechanisms of signal transmission across their synapses suggest they encode very different components of the vestibular input. The slower membrane kinetics and fully quantal mode of transmission onto multiple afferent contacts makes type-II cells suited for the slower, graded representation of head position. The rapid membrane kinetics and presence of a dual mode of, potentially instantaneous, transmission in type-I cells could specialise them for driving the rapid vestibular reflexes.

2.3 Hair cells loss and strategies for restoring auditory function

The loss of hair cells can result from several environmental insults including infectious agents, drugs such as aminoglycoside antibiotics or chemotherapeutics, trauma, loud sounds, a host of genetic factors, or ageing. Since mammalian hair cells do not regenerate, in contrast to those in birds and lower vertebrates (reviewed in [166]), their death produces permanent auditory/vestibular deficit [167, 168]. To date, most studies aimed at regenerating hair cells have focused upon cochlear hair cells. One reason for this is that loss of vestibular hair cells can be, at least partially, compensated by the other senses of vision and proprioception. There are currently three major strategies to restore hair cell function: stem-cell therapy, gene therapy, and molecular therapy (see [169–171]; for recent reviews). There has been an enormous advance in these methods in recent years, that we briefly discuss in the following sections. We refer to some excellent recent reviews on the different areas for those interested in exploring this topic further.

2.3.1 Stem-cell therapies

Stem cells have the potential to self-renew and the ability to differentiate into multiple cell types. It is now well understood that a specific population of resident supporting cells, marked with the stem cell markers Lgr5, Lgr6, Sox2, Sox9, Frizzled-9, EPCAM, and ABCG2 in the organ of Corti, commonly known as cochlear stem/progenitor cells, hold the potential to proliferate and differentiate to form both hair cells and supporting cells (reviewed in [172]). There are two potential stem cell-based approaches that could be used to treat deafness. The first is the stimulation of the resident stem/progenitor cells within the inner ear to proliferate, therefore allowing them to replace the lost hair cells (reviewed in [173]). The basic limitation of this approach is the insufficient number of resident stem/progenitor cells in the inner ear, which means that only a small number of hair cells could potentially be replaced. The second approach is the exogenous supply of stem cells (stem cell transplantation) into the inner ear. The inner ear stem/progenitor cells, also called sensory precursor cells [174], are induced to re-enter the cell cycle by activating the inner ear-related signal pathways. Precursor cell proliferation and differentiation is normally regulated by various signalling pathways, including WNT, Notch, BMP/Smad, FGF, IGF, and Shh pathways [175–178]. The regulation of these pathways is very important for the induction of inner ear precursor cell differentiation into mature hair cells. In a recent review, Waqas et al. [172] discuss the potential for stem cells to combat sensorineural hearing loss in mammals, and explain their current therapeutic applications.

2.3.2 Gene therapies

About fifty percent of inner ear disorders are caused by genetic mutations. Gene therapy is the treatment of diseases using genetic material (DNAs or RNAs). Recent progress in developing gene therapy treatments for genetic hearing loss has demonstrated tantalising proof-of-principle in animal models (see *e.g.*, [179, 180]). In their reviews, Ahmed et al. [181] and Shibata et al. [182] discuss progress, prospects, and challenges for gene therapy in the inner ear. They focus on technical aspects, including routes of gene delivery to the inner ear, choice of vectors, promoters, inner ear targets, therapeutic strategies, preliminary success stories, and points to consider for translating of these successes to the clinic.

2.3.3 Molecular therapies

Pharmacological compounds that could induce generation of new hair cells would be particularly attractive for treating patients with hearing loss caused by hair cell death. A few studies have now reported generation of new hair cells by manipulating endogenous signalling pathways in supporting cells and in hair cells (reviewed in [171, 183]). In short, the differentiation efficiency of inner ear stem/progenitor cells into hair cells remains low. An insufficient number of new hair cells, immature new hair cells without the function of mature hair cells, and long–term survival of new hair cells are all key problems and difficulties that need to be resolved.

3. Conclusions

Mammalian hair cells are exquisite sensory receptors that, over hundreds of millions of years of evolution, have refined strategies to signal sound vibrations or head movements with amazing sensitivity and precision. Despite the notable increase in our knowledge of the mechanisms and molecules involved in hair cell function, there are still several aspects that remain to be elucidated. These include the intimate mechanisms controlling phase-locked quantal release in cochlear IHCs, and the nature of non-quantal transmission in vestibular type-I hair cells, as outlined above. Unfortunately, the complex molecular machinery responsible for sensory transduction and signalling make hair cells highly susceptible to several environmental ototoxic agents, genetic mutation, and ageing. Hair cells loss in mammals is permanent. Although the potential for regenerating hair cells appears to be present in adult mammalian inner ears, it requires their correct integration into an existing, mature organ. The new hair cells will need to be properly positioned in the epithelium according to their specific function (e.g., the hair cell type and location within the sensory epithelium), and properly innervated (*e.g.*, calyx or bouton terminal in the vestibular epithelia). However, precise localization and connectivity may not be an absolute requirement to restore significant functionality. As successful cochlear implants have demonstrated, the central auditory pathways are capable of learning how to interpret an imperfect or incomplete sensory input. The recent explosion of work using gene therapy to restore inner ear function in mouse models represents huge potential for the development future clinical applications for curing auditory and vestibular disorders in humans.

Acknowledgements

All authors contributed equally. The authors thank W. Marcotti (University of Sheffield, UK) for his comments on a previous version of the manuscript.

Conflict of interest

The authors declare no conflict of interest.

Author details

Sergio Masetto[1*], Paolo Spaiardi[2] and Stuart J. Johnson[3]

1 Department of Brain and Behavioural Sciences, University of Pavia, Pavia, Italy

2 Department of Biology and Biotechnology, University of Pavia, Pavia, Italy

3 School of Biosciences, University of Sheffield, Sheffield, UK

*Address all correspondence to: smasetto@unipv.it

References

[1] Marcotti W. Functional assembly of mammalian cochlear hair cells. Experimental Physiology. 2012;**97**(4):438-451. DOI: 10.1113/expphysiol.2011.059303

[2] Kazmierczak P, Sakaguchi H, Tokita J, Wilson-Kubalek EM, Milligan RA, Müller U, et al. Cadherin 23 and protocadherin 15 interact to form tip-link filaments in sensory hair cells. Nature. 2007;**449**(7158):87-91. DOI: 10.1038/nature06091

[3] Corey DP, Akyuz N, Holt JR. Function and dysfunction of TMC channels in inner ear hair cells. Cold Spring Harbor Perspectives in Medicine. 2019;**9**(10):a033506. DOI: 10.1101/cshperspect.a033506

[4] Zheng W, Holt JR. The Mechanosensory transduction machinery in inner ear hair cells. Annual Review of Biophysics. 2021;**50**:31-51. DOI: 10.1146/annurev-biophys-062420-081842. Epub 2020 Dec 7

[5] Kurima K, Peters LM, Yang Y, Riazuddin S, Ahmed ZM, Naz S, et al. Dominant and recessive deafness caused by mutations of a novel gene, TMC1, required for cochlear hair-cell function. Nature Genetics. 2002;**30**(3):277-284. DOI: 10.1038/ng842. Epub 2002 Feb 19

[6] Kawashima Y, Géléoc GS, Kurima K, Labay V, Lelli A, Asai Y, et al. Mechanotransduction in mouse inner ear hair cells requires transmembrane channel-like genes. The Journal of Clinical Investigation. 2011;**121**(12):4796-4809. DOI: 10.1172/JCI60405. Epub 2011 Nov 21

[7] Hudspeth AJ. How hearing happens. Neuron. 1997;**19**(5):947-950. DOI: 10.1016/s0896-6273(00)80385-2

[8] Goldberg JM, Fernandez C. Physiology of peripheral neurons innervating semicircular canals of the squirrel monkey. I. Resting discharge and response to constant angular accelerations. Journal of Neurophysiology. 1971;**34**(4):635-660. DOI: 10.1152/jn.1971.34.4.635

[9] Liberman MC. Auditory-nerve response from cats raised in a low-noise chamber. The Journal of the Acoustical Society of America. 1978;**63**(2):442-455. DOI: 10.1121/1.381736

[10] Bosher SK, Warren RL. Very low calcium content of cochlear endolymph, an extracellular fluid. Nature. 1978;**273**(5661):377-378. DOI: 10.1038/273377a0

[11] Wangemann P. Supporting sensory transduction: Cochlear fluid homeostasis and the endocochlear potential. The Journal of Physiology. 2006;**576**(Pt 1):11-21. DOI: 10.1113/jphysiol.2006.112888. Epub 2006 Jul 20

[12] Ciuman RR. Stria vascularis and vestibular dark cells: Characterisation of main structures responsible for inner-ear homeostasis, and their pathophysiological relations. The Journal of Laryngology and Otology. 2009;**123**(2):151-162. DOI: 10.1017/S0022215108002624. Epub 2008 Jun 23

[13] Von Bekesy G. Resting potentials inside the cochlear partition of the Guinea pig. Nature. 1952;**169**(4293):241-242. DOI: 10.1038/169241a0

[14] Tasaki I. Hearing. Annual Review of Physiology. 1957;**19**:417-438. DOI: 10.1146/annurev.ph.19.030157.002221

[15] Casale J, Agarwal A. Anatomy, head and neck, ear endolymph. In: StatPearls [Internet]. Treasure Island (FL): StatPearls Publishing; 2022. p. 2022

[16] Lysakowski A, Goldberg JM. Ultrastructural analysis of the cristae ampullares in the squirrel monkey (Saimiri sciureus). The Journal of Comparative Neurology. 2008;**511**(1):47-64. DOI: 10.1002/cne.21827

[17] Lenzi D, von Gersdorff H. Structure suggests function: The case for synaptic ribbons as exocytotic nanomachines. BioEssays. 2001;**23**(9):831-840. DOI: 10.1002/bies.1118

[18] Matthews G, Fuchs P. The diverse roles of ribbon synapses in sensory neurotransmission. Nature Reviews. Neuroscience. 2010;**11**(12):812-822. DOI: 10.1038/nrn2924. Epub 2010 Nov 3

[19] Moser T, Grabner CP, Schmitz F. Sensory processing at ribbon synapses in the retina and the cochlea. Physiological Reviews. 2020;**100**(1):103-144. DOI: 10.1152/physrev.00026.2018. Epub 2019 Aug 2

[20] Pangrsic T, Singer JH, Koschak A. Voltage-gated calcium channels: Key players in sensory coding in the retina and the inner ear. Physiological Reviews. 2018;**98**(4):2063-2096. DOI: 10.1152/physrev.00030.2017

[21] Dulon D, Safieddine S, Jones SM, Petit C. Otoferlin is critical for a highly sensitive and linear calcium-dependent exocytosis at vestibular hair cell ribbon synapses. The Journal of Neuroscience. 2009;**29**(34):10474-10487. DOI: 10.1523/JNEUROSCI.1009-09.2009

[22] Glowatzki E, Fuchs PA. Transmitter release at the hair cell ribbon synapse. Nature Neuroscience. 2002;**5**(2):147-154. DOI: 10.1038/nn796

[23] Sadeghi SG, Pyott SJ, Yu Z, Glowatzki E. Glutamatergic signaling at the vestibular hair cell calyx synapse. The Journal of Neuroscience. 2014;**34**(44):14536-14550. DOI: 10.1523/JNEUROSCI.0369-13.2014

[24] Brownell WE, Bader CR, Bertrand D, de Ribaupierre Y. Evoked mechanical responses of isolated cochlear outer hair cells. Science. 1985;**227**(4683):194-196. DOI: 10.1126/science.3966153

[25] Eatock RA. Specializations for fast signaling in the Amniote vestibular inner ear. Integrative and Comparative Biology. 2018;**58**(2):341-350. DOI: 10.1093/icb/icy069

[26] Atkinson PJ, Huarcaya Najarro E, Sayyid ZN, Cheng AG. Sensory hair cell development and regeneration: Similarities and differences. Development. 2015;**142**(9):1561-1571. DOI: 10.1242/dev.114926

[27] Burns JC, Stone JS. Development and regeneration of vestibular hair cells in mammals. Seminars in Cell & Developmental Biology. 2017;**65**:96-105. DOI: 10.1016/j.semcdb.2016.11.001. Epub 2016 Nov 15

[28] Corns LF, Bardhan T, Houston O, et al. Functional development of hair cells in the mammalian inner ear. In: Romand R, Nieto V, editors. Development of Auditory and Vestibular Systems. Ist ed. London: Academic Press; 2014. pp. 155-188. ISBN 9780124080881. DOI: 10.1016/B978-0-12-408088-1.00006-3

[29] Warchol ME, Massoodnia R, Pujol R, Cox BC, Stone JS. Development of hair cell phenotype and calyx nerve terminals in the neonatal mouse utricle. The Journal of Comparative Neurology. 2019;**527**(11):1913-1928. DOI: 10.1002/cne.24658. Epub 2019 Feb 22

[30] Maudoux A, Vitry S, El-Amraoui A. Vestibular deficits in deafness: Clinical presentation, animal modeling, and treatment solutions. Frontiers in Neurology. 2022;**13**:816534. DOI: 10.3389/fneur.2022.816534

[31] Nicolson T. Navigating hereditary hearing loss: Pathology of the inner ear. Frontiers in Cellular Neuroscience. 2021;**15**:660812. DOI: 10.3389/fncel.2021.660812

[32] Florentine M, Buus S, Mason CR. Level discrimination as a function of level for tones from 0.25 to 16 kHz. The Journal of the Acoustical Society of America. 1987;**81**(5):1528-1541. DOI: 10.1121/1.394505

[33] Viemeister NF. Auditory intensity discrimination at high frequencies in the presence of noise. Science. 1983;**221**(4616):1206-1208. DOI: 10.1126/science.6612337

[34] Ruben RJ. The developing concept of Tonotopic Organization of the Inner ear. Journal of the Association for Research in Otolaryngology. 2020;**21**(1):1-20. DOI: 10.1007/s10162-019-00741-3. Epub 2020 Feb 4. Erratum in: J Assoc Res Otolaryngol. 2020;21(2):199

[35] Fettiplace R, Hackney CM. The sensory and motor roles of auditory hair cells. Nature Reviews. Neuroscience. 2006;**7**(1):19-29. DOI: 10.1038/nrn1828

[36] Fettiplace R. Hair cell transduction, tuning, and synaptic transmission in the mammalian cochlea. Comprehensive Physiology. 2017;**7**(4):1197-1227. DOI: 10.1002/cphy.c160049

[37] Ashmore J. Cochlear outer hair cell motility. Physiological Reviews. 2008;**88**(1):173-210. DOI: 10.1152/physrev.00044.2006

[38] Bear MF, Connors BW, Paradiso MA. Neuroscience: Exploring the Brain. 3rd ed. Baltimore, MD: Lippincott Williams & Wilkins; 2006. ISBN 0-7817-6003-8

[39] Cheatham MA, Dallos P. Longitudinal comparisons of IHC ac and dc receptor potentials recorded from the Guinea pig cochlea. Hearing Research. 1993;**68**(1):107-114. DOI: 10.1016/0378-5955(93)90069-d

[40] Dallos P. Response characteristics of mammalian cochlear hair cells. The Journal of Neuroscience. 1985;**5**(6):1591-1608. DOI: 10.1523/JNEUROSCI.05-06-01591.1985

[41] Palmer AR, Russell IJ. Phase-locking in the cochlear nerve of the Guinea-pig and its relation to the receptor potential of inner hair-cells. Hearing Research. 1986;**24**(1):1-15. DOI: 10.1016/0378-5955(86)90002-x

[42] Russell IJ, Sellick PM. Intracellular studies of hair cells in the mammalian cochlea. The Journal of Physiology. 1978;**284**:261-290. DOI: 10.1113/jphysiol.1978.sp012540

[43] Jeng J-Y, Ceriani F, Hendry A, Johnson SL, Yen P, Simmons DD, et al. Hair cell maturation is differentially regulated along the tonotopic axis of the mammalian cochlea. The Journal of Physiology. 2020;**598**(1):151-170. DOI: 10.1113/JP279012. Epub 2019 Dec 21

[44] Platzer J, Engel J, Schrott-Fischer A, Stephan K, Bova S, Chen H, et al. Congenital deafness and sinoatrial node dysfunction in mice lacking class D L-type Ca2+ channels. Cell. 2000;**102**(1):89-97. DOI: 10.1016/s0092-8674(00)00013-1

[45] Brandt A, Striessnig J, Moser T. CaV1.3 channels are essential for development and presynaptic

activity of cochlear inner hair cells. The Journal of Neuroscience. 2003;**23**(34):10832-10840. DOI: 10.1523/JNEUROSCI.23-34-10832.2003

[46] Baig SM, Koschak A, Lieb A, Gebhart M, Dafinger C, Nürnberg G, et al. Loss of Ca(v)1.3 (CACNA1D) function in a human channelopathy with bradycardia and congenital deafness. Nature Neuroscience. 2011;**14**(1):77-84. DOI: 10.1038/nn.2694. Epub 2010 Dec 5

[47] Kros CJ, Ruppersberg JP, Rüsch A. Expression of a potassium current in inner hair cells during development of hearing in mice. Nature. 1998;**394**(6690):281-284. DOI: 10.1038/28401

[48] Marcotti W, Johnson SL, Holley MC, Kros CJ. Developmental changes in the expression of potassium currents of embryonic, neonatal and mature mouse inner hair cells. The Journal of Physiology. 2003;**548**(Pt 2):383-400. DOI: 10.1113/jphysiol.2002.034801. Epub 2003 Feb 14. Erratum in: J Physiol. 2003 Aug 1;550(Pt 3):996

[49] Oliver D, Knipper M, Derst C, Fakler B. Resting potential and submembrane calcium concentration of inner hair cells in the isolated mouse cochlea are set by KCNQ-type potassium channels. The Journal of Neuroscience. 2003;**23**(6):2141-2149. DOI: 10.1523/JNEUROSCI.23-06-02141.2003

[50] Dierich M, Altoè A, Koppelmann J, Evers S, Renigunta V, Schäfer MK, et al. Optimized tuning of auditory inner hair cells to encode complex sound through synergistic activity of six independent K+ current entities. Cell Reports. 2020;**32**(1):107869. DOI: 10.1016/j.celrep.2020.107869

[51] Johnson SL. Membrane properties specialize mammalian inner hair cells for frequency or intensity encoding. eLife. 2015;**4**:e08177. DOI: 10.7554/eLife.08177

[52] Chirila FV, Rowland KC, Thompson JM, Spirou GA. Development of gerbil medial superior olive: Integration of temporally delayed excitation and inhibition at physiological temperature. The Journal of Physiology. 2007;**584**(Pt 1):167-190. DOI: 10.1113/jphysiol.2007.137976. Epub 2007 Aug 9

[53] Caird D, Klinke R. Processing of binaural stimuli by cat superior olivary complex neurons. Experimental Brain Research. 1983;**52**(3):385-399. DOI: 10.1007/BF00238032

[54] Grothe B, Pecka M, McAlpine D. Mechanisms of sound localization in mammals. Physiological Reviews. 2010;**90**(3):983-1012. DOI: 10.1152/physrev.00026.2009

[55] Meyer AC, Frank T, Khimich D, Hoch G, Riedel D, Chapochnikov NM, et al. Tuning of synapse number, structure and function in the cochlea. Nature Neuroscience. 2009;**12**(4):444-453. DOI: 10.1038/nn.2293. Epub 2009 Mar 8

[56] Kiang NY, Rho JM, Northrop CC, Liberman MC, Ryugo DK. Hair-cell innervation by spiral ganglion cells in adult cats. Science. 1982;**217**(4555):175-177. DOI: 10.1126/science.7089553

[57] Pujol R, Lavigne Rebillard M, Lenoir M. Development of sensory and neural structures in the mammalian cochlea. In: Rubel EW, Popper AN, Fay RR, editors. Development of the Auditory System. Springer Handbook of Auditory Research. Vol. XII. New York: Springer; 1997. pp. 146-192

[58] Bulankina AV, Moser T. Neural circuit development in the mammalian cochlea. Physiology (Bethesda, Md.).

2012;**27**(2):100-112. DOI: 10.1152/physiol.00036.2011

[59] Liberman MC. Morphological differences among radial afferent fibers in the cat cochlea: An electron-microscopic study of serial sections. Hearing Research. 1980;**3**(1):45-63. DOI: 10.1016/0378-5955(80)90007-6

[60] Liberman MC, Dodds LW, Pierce S. Afferent and efferent innervation of the cat cochlea: Quantitative analysis with light and electron microscopy. The Journal of Comparative Neurology. 1990;**301**(3):443-460. DOI: 10.1002/cne.903010309. Erratum in: J Comp Neurol 1991 Feb 8;304(2):341

[61] Liberman LD, Wang H, Liberman MC. Opposing gradients of ribbon size and AMPA receptor expression underlie sensitivity differences among cochlear-nerve/hair-cell synapses. The Journal of Neuroscience. 2011;**31**(3):801-808. DOI: 10.1523/JNEUROSCI.3389-10.2011

[62] Schmitz F, Königstorfer A, Südhof TC. RIBEYE, a component of synaptic ribbons: A protein's journey through evolution provides insight into synaptic ribbon function. Neuron. 2000;**28**(3):857-872. DOI: 10.1016/s0896-6273(00)00159-8

[63] Rutherford MA, von Gersdorff H, Goutman JD. Encoding sound in the cochlea: From receptor potential to afferent discharge. The Journal of Physiology. 2021;**599**(10):2527-2557. DOI: 10.1113/JP279189. Epub 2021 Mar 29

[64] Wichmann C, Moser T. Relating structure and function of inner hair cell ribbon synapses. Cell and Tissue Research. 2015;**361**(1):95-114. DOI: 10.1007/s00441-014-2102-7. Epub 2015 Jan 22

[65] Zampini V, Johnson SL, Franz C, Lawrence ND, Münkner S, Engel J, et al. Elementary properties of CaV1.3 Ca(2+) channels expressed in mouse cochlear inner hair cells. The Journal of Physiology. 2010;**588**(Pt 1):187-199. DOI: 10.1113/jphysiol.2009.181917. Epub 2009 Nov 16

[66] Zampini V, Johnson SL, Franz C, Knipper M, Holley MC, Magistretti J, et al. Burst activity and ultrafast activation kinetics of CaV1.3 Ca^{2+} channels support presynaptic activity in adult gerbil hair cell ribbon synapses. The Journal of Physiology. 2013;**591**(16):3811-3820. DOI: 10.1113/jphysiol.2013.251272. Epub 2013 May 27

[67] Zampini V, Johnson SL, Franz C, Knipper M, Holley MC, Magistretti J, et al. Fine tuning of CaV1.3 Ca2+ channel properties in adult inner hair cells positioned in the most sensitive region of the gerbil cochlea. PLoS One. 2014;**9**(11):e113750. DOI: 10.1371/journal.pone.0113750

[68] Johnson SL, Marcotti W. Biophysical properties of CaV1.3 calcium channels in gerbil inner hair cells. The Journal of Physiology. 2008;**586**(4):1029-1042. DOI: 10.1113/jphysiol.2007.145219. Epub 2008 Jan 3

[69] Nouvian R, Neef J, Bulankina AV, Reisinger E, Pangršič T, Frank T, et al. Exocytosis at the hair cell ribbon synapse apparently operates without neuronal SNARE proteins. Nature Neuroscience. 2011;**14**(4):411-413. DOI: 10.1038/nn.2774. Epub 2011 Mar 6

[70] Reisinger E, Bresee C, Neef J, Nair R, Reuter K, Bulankina A, et al. Probing the functional equivalence of otoferlin and synaptotagmin 1 in exocytosis. The Journal of Neuroscience. 2011;**31**(13):4886-4895. DOI: 10.1523/JNEUROSCI.5122-10.2011

[71] Roux I, Safieddine S, Nouvian R, Grati M, Simmler MC, Bahloul A, et al. Otoferlin, defective in a human deafness form, is essential for exocytosis at the auditory ribbon synapse. Cell. 2006;**127**(2):277-289. DOI: 10.1016/j.cell.2006.08.040

[72] Vincent PF, Bouleau Y, Safieddine S, Petit C, Dulon D. Exocytotic machineries of vestibular type I and cochlear ribbon synapses display similar intrinsic otoferlin-dependent Ca2+ sensitivity but a different coupling to Ca2+ channels. The Journal of Neuroscience. 2014;**34**(33):10853-10869. DOI: 10.1523/JNEUROSCI.0947-14.2014

[73] Safieddine S, El-Amraoui A, Petit C. The auditory hair cell ribbon synapse: From assembly to function. Annual Review of Neuroscience. 2012;**35**:509-528. DOI: 10.1146/annurev-neuro-061010-113705

[74] Yasunaga S, Grati M, Cohen-Salmon M, El-Amraoui A, Mustapha M, Salem N, et al. A mutation in OTOF, encoding otoferlin, a FER-1-like protein, causes DFNB9, a nonsyndromic form of deafness. Nature Genetics. 1999;**21**(4):363-369. DOI: 10.1038/7693

[75] Johnson SL, Franz C, Kuhn S, Furness DN, Rüttiger L, Münkner S, et al. Synaptotagmin IV determines the linear Ca2+ dependence of vesicle fusion at auditory ribbon synapses. Nature Neuroscience. 2010;**13**(1):45-52. DOI: 10.1038/nn.2456. Epub 2009 Dec 13

[76] Südhof TC. Synaptotagmins: Why so many? The Journal of Biological Chemistry. 2002;**277**(10):7629-7632. DOI: 10.1074/jbc.R100052200. Epub 2001 Dec 5

[77] Beutner D, Voets T, Neher E, Moser T. Calcium dependence of exocytosis and endocytosis at the cochlear inner hair cell afferent synapse. Neuron. 2001;**29**(3):681-690. DOI: 10.1016/s0896-6273(01)00243-4

[78] Brandt A, Khimich D, Moser T. Few CaV1.3 channels regulate the exocytosis of a synaptic vesicle at the hair cell ribbon synapse. The Journal of Neuroscience. 2005;**25**(50):11577-11585. DOI: 10.1523/JNEUROSCI.3411-05.2005

[79] Johnson SL, Marcotti W, Kros CJ. Increase in efficiency and reduction in Ca2+ dependence of exocytosis during development of mouse inner hair cells. The Journal of Physiology. 2005;**563**(Pt 1):177-191. DOI: 10.1113/jphysiol.2004.074740. Epub 2004 Dec 21

[80] Johnson SL, Forge A, Knipper M, Münkner S, Marcotti W. Tonotopic variation in the calcium dependence of neurotransmitter release and vesicle pool replenishment at mammalian auditory ribbon synapses. The Journal of Neuroscience. 2008;**28**(30):7670-7678. DOI: 10.1523/JNEUROSCI.0785-08.2008

[81] Johnson SL, Olt J, Cho S, von Gersdorff H, Marcotti W. The coupling between Ca2+ channels and the Exocytotic Ca2+ sensor at hair cell ribbon synapses varies Tonotopically along the mature cochlea. The Journal of Neuroscience. 2017;**37**(9):2471-2484. DOI: 10.1523/JNEUROSCI.2867-16.2017. Epub 2017 Feb 2

[82] Moser T, Beutner D. Kinetics of exocytosis and endocytosis at the cochlear inner hair cell afferent synapse of the mouse. Proceedings of the National Academy of Sciences of the United States of America. 2000;**97**(2):883-888. DOI: 10.1073/pnas.97.2.883

[83] Rutherford MA, Pangršič T. Molecular anatomy and physiology of exocytosis in sensory hair cells.

Cell Calcium. 2012;**52**(3-4):327-337. DOI: 10.1016/j.ceca.2012.05.008. Epub 2012 Jun 6

[84] Wong AB, Rutherford MA, Gabrielaitis M, Pangrsic T, Göttfert F, Frank T, et al. Developmental refinement of hair cell synapses tightens the coupling of Ca2+ influx to exocytosis. The EMBO Journal. 2014;**33**(3):247-264. DOI: 10.1002/embj.201387110. Epub 2014 Jan 17

[85] Magistretti J, Spaiardi P, Johnson SL, Masetto S. Elementary properties of Ca(2+) channels and their influence on multivesicular release and phase-locking at auditory hair cell ribbon synapses. Frontiers in Cellular Neuroscience. 2015;**9**:123. DOI: 10.3389/fncel.2015.00123

[86] Matveev V, Bertram R, Sherman A. Calcium cooperativity of exocytosis as a measure of Ca^2+ channel domain overlap. Brain Research. 2011;**1398**:126-138. DOI: 10.1016/j.brainres.2011.05.011. Epub 2011 May 12

[87] Fuchs PA. Time and intensity coding at the hair cell's ribbon synapse. The Journal of Physiology. 2005;**566**(Pt 1):7-12. DOI: 10.1113/jphysiol.2004.082214. Epub 2005 Apr 21

[88] Goutman JD. Transmitter release from cochlear hair cells is phase locked to cyclic stimuli of different intensities and frequencies. The Journal of Neuroscience. 2012;**32**(47):17025-1735a. DOI: 10.1523/JNEUROSCI.0457-12.2012. Erratum in: J Neurosci. 2015 May 13;**35**(19):7654

[89] Li GL, Cho S, von Gersdorff H. Phase-locking precision is enhanced by multiquantal release at an auditory hair cell ribbon synapse. Neuron. 2014;**83**(6):1404-1417. DOI: 10.1016/j.neuron.2014.08.027. Epub 2014 Sep 4

[90] Rose JE, Brugge JF, Anderson DJ, Hind JE. Phase-locked response to low-frequency tones in single auditory nerve fibers of the squirrel monkey. Journal of Neurophysiology. 1967;**30**(4):769-793. DOI: 10.1152/jn.1967.30.4.769

[91] Goutman JD, Glowatzki E. Time course and calcium dependence of transmitter release at a single ribbon synapse. Proceedings of the National Academy of Sciences of the United States of America. 2007;**104**(41):16341-16346. DOI: 10.1073/pnas.0705756104. Epub 2007 Oct 2

[92] Grant L, Yi E, Glowatzki E. Two modes of release shape the postsynaptic response at the inner hair cell ribbon synapse. The Journal of Neuroscience. 2010;**30**(12):4210-4220. DOI: 10.1523/JNEUROSCI.4439-09.2010

[93] Li GL, Keen E, Andor-Ardó D, Hudspeth AJ, von Gersdorff H. The unitary event underlying multiquantal EPSCs at a hair cell's ribbon synapse. The Journal of Neuroscience. 2009;**29**(23):7558-7568. DOI: 10.1523/JNEUROSCI.0514-09.2009

[94] Heil P, Neubauer H, Irvine DR. An improved model for the rate-level functions of auditory-nerve fibers. Journal of Neuroscience. 2011;**31**(43):15424-15437. DOI: 10.1523/JNEUROSCI.1638-11.2011. Erratum in: Journal of Neuroscience. 23 Nov 2011;**31**(47):17326

[95] Ohlemiller KK, Siegel JH. Cochlear basal and apical differences reflected in the effects of cooling on responses of single auditory nerve fibers. Hearing Research. 1994;**80**(2):174-190. DOI: 10.1016/0378-5955(94)90109-0

[96] Johnson SL, Beurg M, Marcotti W, Fettiplace R. Prestin-driven cochlear

amplification is not limited by the outer hair cell membrane time constant. Neuron. 2011;**70**(6):1143-1154. DOI: 10.1016/j.neuron.2011.04.024

[97] Kharkovets T, Dedek K, Maier H, Schweizer M, Khimich D, Nouvian R, et al. Mice with altered KCNQ4 K+ channels implicate sensory outer hair cells in human progressive deafness. The EMBO Journal. 2006;**25**(3):642-652. DOI: 10.1038/sj.emboj.7600951. Epub 2006 Jan 26

[98] Kubisch C, Schroeder BC, Friedrich T, Lütjohann B, El-Amraoui A, Marlin S, et al. KCNQ4, a novel potassium channel expressed in sensory outer hair cells, is mutated in dominant deafness. Cell. 1999;**96**(3):437-446. DOI: 10.1016/s0092-8674(00)80556-5

[99] Marcotti W, Kros CJ. Developmental expression of the potassium current IK,n contributes to maturation of mouse outer hair cells. The Journal of Physiology. 1999;**520**(Pt 3):653-660. DOI: 10.1111/j.1469-7793.1999.00653.x

[100] Mammano F, Ashmore JF. Differential expression of outer hair cell potassium currents in the isolated cochlea of the Guinea-pig. The Journal of Physiology. 1996;**496**(Pt 3):639-646. DOI: 10.1113/jphysiol.1996.sp021715

[101] Ceriani F, Hendry A, Jeng JY, Johnson SL, Stephani F, Olt J, Holley MC, Mammano F, Engel J, Kros CJ, Simmons DD, Marcotti W. Coordinated calcium signalling in cochlear sensory and non-sensory cells refines afferent innervation of outer hair cells. The EMBO Journal. 2019;**38**(9):e99839. DOI: 10.15252/embj.201899839. Epub 2019 Feb 25.

[102] Michna M, Knirsch M, Hoda JC, Muenkner S, Langer P, Platzer J, et al. Cav1.3 (alpha1D) Ca2+ currents in neonatal outer hair cells of mice. The Journal of Physiology. 2003;**553**(Pt 3):747-758. DOI: 10.1113/jphysiol.2003.053256. Epub 2003 Sep 26

[103] Knirsch M, Brandt N, Braig C, Kuhn S, Hirt B, Münkner S, et al. Persistence of Ca(v)1.3 Ca2+ channels in mature outer hair cells supports outer hair cell afferent signaling. The Journal of Neuroscience. 2007;**27**(24):6442-6451. DOI: 10.1523/JNEUROSCI.5364-06.2007

[104] Moglie MJ, Wengier DL, Elgoyhen AB, Goutman JD. Synaptic contributions to Cochlear outer hair cell Ca2+ dynamics. The Journal of Neuroscience. 2021;**41**(32):6812-6821. DOI: 10.1523/JNEUROSCI.3008-20.2021. Epub 2021 Jul 12

[105] Wood MB, Nowak N, Mull K, Goldring A, Lehar M, Fuchs PA. Acoustic trauma increases ribbon number and size in outer hair cells of the mouse cochlea. Journal of the Association for Research in Otolaryngology. 2021;**22**(1):19-31. DOI: 10.1007/s10162-020-00777-w. Epub 2020 Nov 5

[106] Zheng J, Shen W, He DZ, Long KB, Madison LD, Dallos P. Prestin is the motor protein of cochlear outer hair cells. Nature. 2000;**405**(6783):149-155. DOI: 10.1038/35012009

[107] Schaechinger TJ, Oliver D. Nonmammalian orthologs of prestin (SLC26A5) are electrogenic divalent/chloride anion exchangers. Proceedings of the National Academy of Sciences of the United States of America. 2007;**104**(18):7693-7698. DOI: 10.1073/pnas.0608583104. Epub 2007 Apr 18

[108] He DZ, Jia S, Sato T, Zuo J, Andrade LR, Riordan GP, et al. Changes in plasma membrane structure and electromotile properties in prestin deficient

outer hair cells. Cytoskeleton (Hoboken). 2010;**67**(1):43-55. DOI: 10.1002/cm.20423

[109] Liberman MC, Gao J, He DZ, Wu X, Jia S, Zuo J. Prestin is required for electromotility of the outer hair cell and for the cochlear amplifier. Nature. 2002;**419**(6904):300-304. DOI: 10.1038/nature01059. Epub 2002 Aug 28

[110] Liu XZ, Ouyang XM, Xia XJ, Zheng J, Pandya A, Li F, et al. Prestin, a cochlear motor protein, is defective in non-syndromic hearing loss. Human Molecular Genetics. 2003;**12**(10):1155-1162. DOI: 10.1093/hmg/ddg127

[111] Weisz CJC, Lehar M, Hiel H, Glowatzki E, Fuchs PA. Synaptic transfer from outer hair cells to type II afferent fibers in the rat cochlea. The Journal of Neuroscience. 2012;**32**(28):9528-9536. DOI: 10.1523/JNEUROSCI.6194-11.2012

[112] Berglund AM, Ryugo DK. Hair cell innervation by spiral ganglion neurons in the mouse. The Journal of Comparative Neurology. 1987;**255**(4):560-570. DOI: 10.1002/cne.902550408

[113] Weisz CJC, Glowatzki E, Fuchs P. The postsynaptic function of type II cochlear afferents. Nature. 2009;**461**(7267):1126-1129. DOI: 10.1038/nature08487

[114] Weisz CJC, Glowatzki E, Fuchs PA. Excitability of type II cochlear afferents. The Journal of Neuroscience. 2014;**34**(6):2365-2373. DOI: 10.1523/JNEUROSCI.3428-13.2014

[115] Flores EN, Duggan A, Madathany T, Hogan AK, Márquez FG, Kumar G, et al. A non-canonical pathway from cochlea to brain signals tissue-damaging noise. Current Biology. 2015;**25**(5):606-612. DOI: 10.1016/j.cub.2015.01.009. Epub 2015 Jan 29

[116] Liu C, Glowatzki E, Fuchs PA. Unmyelinated type II afferent neurons report cochlear damage. Proceedings of the National Academy of Sciences of the United States of America. 2015;**112**(47):14723-14727. DOI: 10.1073/pnas.1515228112. Epub 2015 Nov 9

[117] Weisz CJC, Williams SG, Eckard CS, Divito CB, Ferreira DW, Fantetti KN, et al. Outer hair cell glutamate signaling through type II spiral ganglion afferents activates neurons in the Cochlear nucleus in response to nondamaging sounds. The Journal of Neuroscience. 2021;**41**(13):2930-2943. DOI: 10.1523/JNEUROSCI.0619-20.2021. Epub 2021 Feb 11

[118] Maison SF, Adams JC, Liberman MC. Olivocochlear innervation in the mouse: Immunocytochemical maps, crossed versus uncrossed contributions, and transmitter colocalization. The Journal of Comparative Neurology. 2003;**455**(3):406-416. DOI: 10.1002/cne.10490

[119] Guinan JJ. Physiology of the medial and lateral Olivocochlear systems. In: Ryugo D, Fay R, editors. Auditory and Vestibular Efferents. Springer Handbook of Auditory Research. Vol. 38. New York, NY: Springer; 2011. DOI: 10.1007/978-1-4419-7070-1_3

[120] Elgoyhen AB, Johnson DS, Boulter J, Vetter DE, Heinemann S. Alpha 9: An acetylcholine receptor with novel pharmacological properties expressed in rat cochlear hair cells. Cell. 1994;**79**(4):705-715. DOI: 10.1016/0092-8674(94)90555-x

[121] Elgoyhen AB, Vetter DE, Katz E, Rothlin CV, Heinemann SF, Boulter J. alpha10: A determinant of nicotinic cholinergic receptor function in mammalian vestibular and cochlear

mechanosensory hair cells. Proceedings of the National Academy of Sciences of the United States of America. 2001;**98**(6):3501-3506. DOI: 10.1073/pnas.051622798. Epub 2001 Mar 6

[122] Oliver D, Klöcker N, Schuck J, Baukrowitz T, Ruppersberg JP, Fakler B. Gating of Ca2+–activated K+ channels controls fast inhibitory synaptic transmission at auditory outer hair cells. Neuron. 2000;**26**(3):595-601. DOI: 10.1016/s0896-6273(00)81197-6

[123] Eatock RA, Songer JE. Vestibular hair cells and afferents: Two channels for head motion signals. Annual Review of Neuroscience. 2011;**34**:501-534. DOI: 10.1146/annurev-neuro-061010-113710

[124] Goldberg JM. Afferent diversity and the organization of central vestibular pathways. Experimental Brain Research. 2000;**130**(3):277-297. DOI: 10.1007/s002210050033

[125] Gulley RL, Bagger-Sjöbäck D. Freeze-fracture studies on the synapse between the type I hair cell and the calyceal terminal in the Guinea-pig vestibular system. Journal of Neurocytology. 1979;**8**(5):591-603. DOI: 10.1007/BF01208511

[126] Lysakowski A, Goldberg JM. A regional ultrastructural analysis of the cellular and synaptic architecture in the chinchilla cristae ampullares. The Journal of Comparative Neurology. 1997;**389**(3):419-443. DOI: 10.1002/(sici)1096-9861(19971222)389:3<419::aid-cne5>3.0.co;2-3

[127] Wersäll J. Studies on the structure and innervation of the sensory epithelium of the cristae ampulares in the Guinea pig; a light and electron microscopic investigation. Acta Oto-Laryngologica. Supplementum. 1956;**126**:1-85

[128] Dieterich M, Brandt T. Vestibulo-ocular reflex. Current Opinion in Neurology. 1995;**8**(1):83-88. DOI: 10.1097/00019052-199502000-00014

[129] Angelaki DE, Cullen KE. Vestibular system: The many facets of a multimodal sense. Annual Review of Neuroscience. 2008;**31**:125-150. DOI: 10.1146/annurev.neuro.31.060407.125555

[130] Kremmyda O, Hüfner K, Flanagin VL, Hamilton DA, Linn J, Strupp M, et al. Beyond dizziness: Virtual navigation, spatial anxiety and hippocampal volume in bilateral Vestibulopathy. Frontiers in Human Neuroscience. 2016;**10**:139. DOI: 10.3389/fnhum.2016.00139

[131] Yoder RM, Taube JS. The vestibular contribution to the head direction signal and navigation. Frontiers in Integrative Neuroscience. 2014;**8**:32. DOI: 10.3389/fnint.2014.00032

[132] Fernandez C, Goldberg JM. Physiology of peripheral neurons innervating semicircular canals of the squirrel monkey. II. Response to sinusoidal stimulation and dynamics of peripheral vestibular system. Journal of Neurophysiology. 1971;**34**(4):661-675. DOI: 10.1152/jn.1971.34.4.661

[133] Ramachandran R, Lisberger SG. Transformation of vestibular signals into motor commands in the vestibuloocular reflex pathways of monkeys. Journal of Neurophysiology. 2006;**96**(3):1061-1074. DOI: 10.1152/jn.00281.2006. Epub 2006 Jun 7

[134] Baird RA, Desmadryl G, Fernández C, Goldberg JM. The vestibular nerve of the chinchilla. II. Relation between afferent response properties and peripheral innervation patterns in the semicircular canals. Journal of Neurophysiology.

1988;**60**(1):182-203. DOI: 10.1152/jn.1988.60.1.182

[135] Goldberg JM, Lysakowski A, Fernández C. Morphophysiological and ultrastructural studies in the mammalian cristae ampullares. Hearing Research. 1990;**49**(1-3):89-102. DOI: 10.1016/0378-5955(90)90097-9

[136] Fernández C, Goldberg JM, Baird RA. The vestibular nerve of the chinchilla. III. Peripheral innervation patterns in the utricular macula. Journal of Neurophysiology. 1990;**63**(4):767-780. DOI: 10.1152/jn.1990.63.4.767

[137] Songer JE, Eatock RA. Tuning and timing in mammalian type I hair cells and calyceal synapses. The Journal of Neuroscience. 2013;**33**(8):3706-3724. DOI: 10.1523/JNEUROSCI.4067-12.2013

[138] Vollrath MA, Eatock RA. Time course and extent of mechanotransducer adaptation in mouse utricular hair cells: Comparison with frog saccular hair cells. Journal of Neurophysiology. 2003;**90**(4):2676-2689. DOI: 10.1152/jn.00893.2002

[139] Bao H, Wong WH, Goldberg JM, Eatock RA. Voltage-gated calcium channel currents in type I and type II hair cells isolated from the rat crista. Journal of Neurophysiology. 2003;**90**(1):155-164. DOI: 10.1152/jn.00244.2003. Erratum in: J Neurophysiol. 2004;91(1):589

[140] Meredith FL, Rennie KJ. Channeling your inner ear potassium: K(+) channels in vestibular hair cells. Hearing Research. 2016;**338**:40-51. DOI: 10.1016/j.heares.2016.01.015. Epub 2016 Feb 4

[141] Rüsch A, Lysakowski A, Eatock RA. Postnatal development of type I and type II hair cells in the mouse utricle: Acquisition of voltage-gated conductances and differentiated morphology. The Journal of Neuroscience. 1998;**18**(18):7487-7501. DOI: 10.1523/JNEUROSCI.18-18-07487.1998

[142] Rennie KJ, Correia MJ. Potassium currents in mammalian and avian isolated type I semicircular canal hair cells. Journal of Neurophysiology. 1994;**71**(1):317-329. DOI: 10.1152/jn.1994.71.1.317

[143] Rüsch A, Eatock RA. A delayed rectifier conductance in type I hair cells of the mouse utricle. Journal of Neurophysiology. 1996;**76**(2):995-1004. DOI: 10.1152/jn.1996.76.2.995

[144] Spaiardi P, Tavazzani E, Manca M, Milesi V, Russo G, Prigioni I, et al. An allosteric gating model recapitulates the biophysical properties of IK,L expressed in mouse vestibular type I hair cells. The Journal of Physiology. 2017;**595**(21):6735-6750. DOI: 10.1113/JP274202. Epub 2017 Sep 24

[145] Hurley KM, Gaboyard S, Zhong M, Price SD, Wooltorton JR, Lysakowski A, et al. M-like K+ currents in type I hair cells and calyx afferent endings of the developing rat utricle. The Journal of Neuroscience. 2006;**26**(40):10253-10269. DOI: 10.1523/JNEUROSCI.2596-06.2006

[146] Contini D, Zampini V, Tavazzani E, Magistretti J, Russo G, Prigioni I, et al. Intercellular K^+ accumulation depolarizes type I vestibular hair cells and their associated afferent nerve calyx. Neuroscience. 2012;**227**:232-246. DOI: 10.1016/j.neuroscience.2012.09.051. Epub 2012 Sep 29

[147] Tavazzani E, Spaiardi P, Zampini V, Contini D, Manca M, Russo G, et al. Distinct roles of Eps8 in the maturation of cochlear and vestibular hair cells. Neuroscience. 2016;**328**:80-91. DOI: 10.1016/j.neuroscience.2016.04.038. Epub 2016 Apr 27

[148] Contini D, Holstein GR, Art JJ. Simultaneous dual recordings from vestibular hair cells and their calyx afferents demonstrate multiple modes of transmission at these specialized endings. Frontiers in Neurology. 2022;**13**:891536. DOI: 10.3389/fneur.2022.891536

[149] Mukhopadhyay M, Pangrsic T. Synaptic transmission at the vestibular hair cells of amniotes. Molecular and Cellular Neurosciences. 2022;**121**:103749. DOI: 10.1016/j.mcn.2022.103749. Epub 2022 Jun 3

[150] Demêmes D, Lleixa A, Dechesne CJ. Cellular and subcellular localization of AMPA-selective glutamate receptors in the mammalian peripheral vestibular system. Brain Research. 1995;**671**(1):83-94. DOI: 10.1016/0006-8993(94)01322-9

[151] Kirk ME, Meredith FL, Benke TA, Rennie KJ. AMPA receptor-mediated rapid EPSCs in vestibular calyx afferents. Journal of Neurophysiology. 2017;**117**(6):2312-2323. DOI: 10.1152/jn.00394.2016. Epub 2017 Mar 15

[152] Manca M, Yen P, Spaiardi P, Russo G, Giunta R, Johnson SL, et al. Current response in Ca V 1.3−/− mouse vestibular and Cochlear hair cells. Frontiers in Neuroscience. 2021;**15**:749483. DOI: 10.3389/fnins.2021.749483

[153] Spaiardi P, Marcotti W, Masetto S, Johnson SL. Signal transmission in mature mammalian vestibular hair cells. Frontiers in Cellular Neuroscience. 2022;**16**:806913. DOI: 10.3389/fncel.2022.806913

[154] Spaiardi P, Marcotti W, Masetto S, Johnson SL. Exocytosis in mouse vestibular type II hair cells shows a high-order Ca2+ dependence that is independent of synaptotagmin-4. Physiological Reports. 2020;**8**(14):e14509. DOI: 10.14814/phy2.14509

[155] Spaiardi P, Tavazzani E, Manca M, Russo G, Prigioni I, Biella G, et al. K+ accumulation and clearance in the calyx synaptic cleft of type I mouse vestibular hair cells. Neuroscience. 2020;**426**:69-86. DOI: 10.1016/j.neuroscience.2019.11.028. Epub 2019 Dec 14

[156] Grossman GE, Leigh RJ, Abel LA, Lanska DJ, Thurston SE. Frequency and velocity of rotational head perturbations during locomotion. Experimental Brain Research. 1988;**70**(3):470-476. DOI: 10.1007/BF00247595

[157] Dou H, Vazquez AE, Namkung Y, Chu H, Cardell EL, Nie L, et al. Null mutation of alpha1D Ca2+ channel gene results in deafness but no vestibular defect in mice. Journal of the Association for Research in Otolaryngology. 2004;**5**(2):215-226. DOI: 10.1007/s10162-003-4020-3

[158] Contini D, Price SD, Art JJ. Accumulation of K+ in the synaptic cleft modulates activity by influencing both vestibular hair cell and calyx afferent in the turtle. The Journal of Physiology. 2017;**595**(3):777-803. DOI: 10.1113/JP273060. Epub 2016 Nov 4

[159] Contini D, Holstein GR, Art JJ. Synaptic cleft microenvironment influences potassium permeation and synaptic transmission in hair cells surrounded by calyx afferents in the turtle. The Journal of Physiology. 2020;**598**(4):853-889. DOI: 10.1113/JP278680. Epub 2019 Nov 29

[160] Holt JC, Chatlani S, Lysakowski A, Goldberg JM. Quantal and nonquantal transmission in calyx-bearing fibers of the turtle posterior crista. Journal of Neurophysiology. 2007;**98**(3):1083-1101. DOI: 10.1152/jn.00332.2007. Epub 2007 Jun 27

[161] Yamashita M, Ohmori H. Synaptic responses to mechanical stimulation in calyceal and Bouton type vestibular afferents studied in an isolated preparation of semicircular canal ampullae of chicken. Experimental Brain Research. 1990;**80**(3):475-488. DOI: 10.1007/BF00227989

[162] Lim R, Kindig AE, Donne SW, Callister RJ, Brichta AM. Potassium accumulation between type I hair cells and calyx terminals in mouse crista. Experimental Brain Research. 2011;**210**(3-4):607-621. DOI: 10.1007/s00221-011-2592-4. Epub 2011 Feb 25

[163] Vroman R, Klaassen LJ, Kamermans M. Ephaptic communication in the vertebrate retina. Frontiers in Human Neuroscience. 2013;**7**:612. DOI: 10.3389/fnhum.2013.00612

[164] Curthoys IS, Burgess AM, Goonetilleke SC. Phase-locking of irregular Guinea pig primary vestibular afferents to high frequency (>250 Hz) sound and vibration. Hearing Research. 2019;**373**:59-70. DOI: 10.1016/j.heares.2018.12.009. Epub 2018 Dec 24. Erratum in: Hear Res. 2020;389:107909

[165] Huterer M, Cullen KE. Vestibuloocular reflex dynamics during high-frequency and high-acceleration rotations of the head on body in rhesus monkey. Journal of Neurophysiology. 2002;**88**(1):13-28. DOI: 10.1152/jn.2002.88.1.13

[166] Rubel EW, Furrer SA, Stone JS. A brief history of hair cell regeneration research and speculations on the future. Hearing Research. 2013;**297**:42-51. DOI: 10.1016/j.heares.2012.12.014. Epub 2013 Jan 12

[167] González-Garrido A, Pujol R, López-Ramírez O, Finkbeiner C, Eatock RA, Stone JS. The differentiation status of hair cells that regenerate naturally in the vestibular inner ear of the adult mouse. The Journal of Neuroscience. 2021;**41**(37):7779-7796. DOI: 10.1523/JNEUROSCI.3127-20.2021. Epub 2021 Jul 23

[168] Groves AK. The challenge of hair cell regeneration. Experimental Biology and Medicine (Maywood, N.J.). 2010;**235**(4):434-446. DOI: 10.1258/ebm.2009.009281

[169] Delmaghani S, El-Amraoui A. J. Inner ear gene therapies take off: Current promises and future challenges. Clinical Medicine 2020;**9**(7):2309. DOI: 10.3390/jcm9072309.

[170] Nacher-Soler G, Garrido JM, Rodríguez-Serrano F. Hearing regeneration and regenerative medicine: Present and future approaches. Archives of Medical Science. 2019;**15**(4):957-967. DOI: 10.5114/aoms.2019.86062. Epub 2019 Jun 20

[171] Xu S, Yang N. Research Progress on the mechanism of Cochlear hair cell regeneration. Frontiers in Cellular Neuroscience. 2021;**15**:732507. DOI: 10.3389/fncel.2021.732507

[172] Waqas M, Us-Salam I, Bibi Z, Wang Y, Li H, Zhu Z, et al. Stem cell-based therapeutic approaches to restore sensorineural hearing loss in mammals. Neural Plasticity. 2020;**2020**:8829660. DOI: 10.1155/2020/8829660

[173] Durán-Alonso MB. Stem cell-based approaches: Possible route to hearing restoration? World Journal of Stem Cells. 2020;**12**(6):422-437. DOI: 10.4252/wjsc.v12.i6.422

[174] Monzack EL, Cunningham LL. Lead roles for supporting actors: Critical functions of inner ear supporting cells. Hearing Research. 2013;**303**:20-29.

DOI: 10.1016/j.heares.2013.01.008. Epub 2013 Jan 21

[175] Munnamalai V, Fekete DM. Notch-Wnt-bmp crosstalk regulates radial patterning in the mouse cochlea in a spatiotemporal manner. Development. 2016;**143**(21):4003-4015. DOI: 10.1242/dev.139469. Epub 2016 Sep 15

[176] Schimmang T. Expression and functions of FGF ligands during early otic development. The International Journal of Developmental Biology. 2007;**51**(6-7):473-481. DOI: 10.1387/ijdb.072334ts

[177] Waqas M, Zhang S, He Z, Tang M, Chai R. Role of Wnt and notch signaling in regulating hair cell regeneration in the cochlea. Frontiers in Medicine. 2016;**10**(3):237-249. DOI: 10.1007/s11684-016-0464-9. Epub 2016 Sep 7

[178] Wu J, Li W, Lin C, Chen Y, Cheng C, Sun S, et al. Co-regulation of the notch and Wnt signaling pathways promotes supporting cell proliferation and hair cell regeneration in mouse utricles. Scientific Reports. 2016;**6**:29418. DOI: 10.1038/srep29418

[179] Jeng J-Y, Carlton AJ, Goodyear RJ, Chinowsky C, Ceriani F, Johnson SL, et al. AAV-mediated rescue of Eps8 expression in vivo restores hair-cell function in a mouse model of recessive deafness. Molecular Therapy—Methods and Clinical Developments. 2022;**26**:355-370. DOI: 10.1016/j.omtm.2022.07.012. eCollection 2022 Sep 8

[180] Nist-Lund CA, Pan B, Patterson A, Asai Y, Chen T, Zhou W, et al. Improved TMC1 gene therapy restores hearing and balance in mice with genetic inner ear disorders. Nature Communications. 2019;**10**(1):236. DOI: 10.1038/s41467-018-08264-w. Erratum in: Nat Commun. 2019 Feb 8;10(1):734

[181] Ahmed H, Shubina-Oleinik O, Holt JR. Emerging gene therapies for genetic hearing loss. Journal of the Association for Research in Otolaryngology. 2017;**18**(5):649-670. DOI: 10.1007/s10162-017-0634-8. Epub 2017 Aug 16

[182] Shibata SB, West MB, Du X, Iwasa Y, Raphael Y, Kopke RD. Gene therapy for hair cell regeneration: Review and new data. Hearing Research. 2020;**394**:107981. DOI: 10.1016/j.heares.2020.107981. Epub 2020 May 5

[183] Géléoc GS, Holt JR. Sound strategies for hearing restoration. Science. 2014;**344**(6184):1241062. DOI: 10.1126/science.1241062

Section 2

Updates on the Diagnosis and Therapy

Chapter 4

Vestibular Therapy

Madalina Georgescu

Abstract

Vestibular therapy is a common topic in physicians' search for updated clinical practice. Early and appropriate vestibular rehabilitation makes a difference in a patient's outcome. Peripheral vestibular impairments are often unilateral and heterogeneous. For this reason, treatment differs depending on the etiology, the moment from the onset, and the age of the patient. Following issues will be addressed in this chapter: medical treatment in the acute phase and subacute/chronic phase of unilateral vestibular loss; repositioning maneuvers for different types of BPPV; vestibular rehabilitation individualized programs, for vestibular neuritis, otolith dysfunction, visual vertigo, bilateral vestibular loss; virtual reality in vestibular rehabilitation programs; evaluation of vestibular rehabilitation programs; and new research treatment options—vibrotactile Balance Bely and vestibular implant.

Keywords: vertigo, peripheral vestibular loss, repositioning maneuvers, vestibular rehabilitation, virtual reality, Balance Belt, vestibular implant

1. Introduction

Vestibular lesions have a noticeable impact on patient's quality of life. Depending on the disease itself, but also on the patient's psychological status, vestibular impairment has severe long-term functional consequences in many cases. After headache, vertigo is one of the most frequent presenting symptoms to physicians in many disciplines, with a lifetime prevalence of almost 30% [1].

Dizziness is a pathologic condition that includes disorders of spatial orientation and motion perception and disturbances in gaze stability, posture, and gait. About 5% of the general population has dizziness, vertigo, or disequilibrium and their prevalence, frequency, and severity increases, in general, with age [2]. It is considered that half of the patients with dizziness have a vestibular dysfunction and in those in whom vestibular lesion is symptomatic, the odds of falling are 12-fold greater [3].

Four out of five patients report severe impairment of daily activities. This is an important issue to address when we talk about vestibular therapy and its benefit for the patient, but also is a parameter which expresses the economic burden of vestibular diseases: absenteeism, high use of health care, and increased risk of fall with its consequences (e.g., hip fracture in elderly).

Dizziness is the main reason for physician appointments in patients over 75 years of age and represents a significant risk factor for falls. Falls are considered the leading cause of serious injury and death in elderly—10% of hospitalization and 50% of accidental deaths.

For all medical, psychological, and economical reasons, vestibular therapy should have appropriate time-course customization, based on the phase of the disease (acute or chronic) and type of the peripheral vestibular pathology (single episode, recurrent episodes), and etiology, if possible (BPPV, vestibular neuritis, endolymphatic hydrops, labyrinthitis, vestibular paroxysmia, third window syndrome, or bilateral vestibular loss). Once the diagnosis is established, a correct drug with appropriate dosage and sufficient duration should be considered. Too low or too high initial dose might be ineffective or not well tolerated. Also, duration is important for better recovery—prolonged antivertiginous agents delay vestibular compensation phenomenon, and diseases such as Menière disease and vestibular migraine require long-term treatment [4].

Treatment management must take into account the natural recovery of a unilateral peripheral vestibular deficit (UVL), through the central vestibular compensation process. This represents a neuroplasticity model of recovery after a UVL, with the highest intensity in the first week after vestibular injury and continues slowly over a long period of time (1 year) [5]. It is an imperfect and incomplete (high acceleration or velocity head movements are not always compensated) phenomenon. Central vestibular compensation must be enhanced and accelerated for the best outcome for the patient, in the shortest possible period of time. This can be obtained with prolonged treatment (at least 3 months) with betahistine associated with vestibular rehabilitation physical programs, bimodal management widely accepted [6–9].

Vestibular rehabilitation (VR) program is based on physical exercises specially designed to overcome imbalance issues and minimize the negative consequences of vestibular impairment, by creating new cortical models of reaction to daily balance challenges.

VR exercises target a reset of the brain through habituation (reduces avoidance of certain positions), adaptation (teaching the unaffected balance receptors to undertake the function of destroyed ones), and substitution (teaching other sensory systems to compensate for the vestibular impairment) strategies. The treatment is focused on improving clear vision when moving the head, reducing the intolerance to movement by use of repetitive eye, head, and body movement, and relearning of balance.

Central compensation of dynamic symptoms involves multiple processes:

- Restoration of peripheral function.
- Compensatory readjustments of brainstem vestibular processing.
- Sensorial substitution of the impaired vestibular function by other sensorial systems (visual and somatosensorial)—use of smooth pursuit instead of the nonfunctional vestibulocular reflex (VOR), for example.
- Functional substitution—use of alternative strategies, with different effectors than the damaged vestibular ones: prediction, saccades instead of VOR, or extensive use of cervical inputs.
- Behavioral changes in order to minimize vestibular challenges and demands.

All above-mentioned processes except the first one (restoration of peripheral function) act competitively: all start simultaneously and act redundantly but using one of them may eliminate the need for others. This selection of the main central compensation process is one of the explanations for variable outcomes of the same process in different patients—dependence on visual substitution impedes upon somatosensorial substitution mechanisms and vice versa.

Customized vestibular rehabilitation programs might diminish this limit of the natural recovery phenomena [10–15], as well as specific drug therapy [16]. The overall outcome of the central compensation process is also influenced by its delay in action. There is a critical period when neuroplasticity of the vestibular central structures is highest (first month after the acute injury) and patients must take advantage of this time-window opportunity in order to trigger early recovery mechanisms [17, 18].

Vestibular rehabilitation exercises may include specific movements which will trigger the symptoms, in order to "desensitize" the vestibular system (habituation) for positional or motion-provoked symptoms and progressively improve the gain of the vestibular reflexes (adaptation). Substitution phenomenon also occurs in order to replace the vestibular lost function through other senses involved in stabilizing gaze, stance, and equilibrium. Besides alternation of the sensory inputs, prediction and anticipation strategies can be implemented. For example, when vestibulo-ocular reflex is impaired, visual stability is obtained through cervical-ocular reflex.

Coordinating learning strategies in order to maximize adaptation and motor learning and avoid overstimulation is very important as well [19].

2. Treatment management of peripheral vestibular dysfunction

Management of a peripheral vestibular syndrome includes often combined vestibular therapies—medication, repositioning maneuvers, vestibular rehabilitation, psychotherapeutic measures or, rarely, surgery and should be customized to the individual particularities of each patient.

This will be the issue to address in the following pages.

2.1 Medical treatment

Anatomical connections between vestibular nuclei and autonomous system explain symptoms associated with a peripheral vestibular lesion:

- Nausea and vomiting
- Pale
- Cold sweating
- Respiratory and circulatory disturbances

All these symptoms appear due to the functional asymmetry of the vestibular nuclei, which receive different information from the inner ear vestibular receptors and the treatment target is to restore the balance between the vestibular nuclei. To achieve this goal, the acute stage treatment implies:

- Sedation of the vestibular system in order to "silence" the difference in activity.
- Reduction and elimination of the autonomous symptoms.

2.1.1 Symptomatic pharmacotherapy: for the first 1: 3 days

Prolonged use impedes central vestibular compensation, a vital process for a good recovery of the vestibular deficit.

1. Targeting the vestibular neurotransmitters:

    a. Cholinergic: anticholinergic drugs = scopolamine, meclizine. They inhibit stimulation (excessive impulses) from the peripheral organs and vestibular nerve and inhibit transmission in the lateral vestibular nucleus. Are contraindicated in high blood pressure and closed angle glaucoma and have important adverse reactions—dry mouth, dilated pupils, urinary retention, sedation, constipation, and confusion.

    b. Histaminergic: antihistaminergic drugs = dimenhydrinate. Its mechanism is uncertain, but it has a central effect by blocking H1 receptors and inhibiting synaptic transmission on medial vestibular nucleus.

    c. GABA neurotransmitters: GABA-ergic drugs = lorazepam, valium. They provoke a central suppression of the vestibular response, reduce anxiety, and also have a sedative and hypnotic effect. They impair central vestibular compensation, and this is the reason they should be administered for at most 3 days. As side effects, impaired memory and addiction should be known.

2. Targeting the vomiting center transmitters:

    a. Dopaminergic (selective dopamine D2 antagonist) = droperidol, has a low incidence of extrapyramidal effects, antiemetic action, improved blood flow, mucosal secretion in GI, antivertigo, anti-migraine headache, and antidepressant activity (in low doses).

    b. Histaminergic (H1).

    c. Serotoninergic (5-HT3 antagonist/5 hydroxytryptamine subtype 3 receptor)—Ondensetron/granisetron, less effective for vestibular emesis and has a high cost.

Other drugs might also be used in the acute phase, such as:

- Calcium channel blockers = Flurnarazine/Cinnarazine
    - vestibular suppression on Ca channel in hair cells
    - antihistamines and anticholinergic activity
    - side effects: sedation, weight gain, Parkinsonism
- Sodium channel blockers = Phenytoin/nerontin/tegretol
    - affect GABA neurotransmitters; glutamate antagonist

- induce central nystagmus
- uncertain mechanism

- Histamine agonists (H1/H3—receptors agonist) = Betahistine
  - increase circulation to the inner ear
  - suppress vestibular function on the healthy side
  - facilitate central vestibular compensation
  - side effects: nausea, headache
  - caution: peptic ulcer, pheochromocytoma
- Acetyl-leucine
  - vestibular suppressant
  - rapid antivertigo effect (IV)

2.1.2 Etiologic-based treatment

General medical treatment mentioned above is associated with an etiological therapy when etiology of the peripheral vestibular deficit is known.

- Steroids—for vestibular neuritis and Menière disease; reduce the duration of vertigo episodes.
  - methylprednisolone 100 mg/day, doses tapered by 20 mg every fourth day within 3 days of symptom onset has a significant effect in improving the recovery of peripheral vestibular function [5].
  - intratympanic corticosteroids—repeated series of weekly injections of 10 mg/ml dexamethasone for 1 month reduce vertigo spells in 48% of patients, without deterioration of auditory hair cells (preserved transient otoacoustic emissions) [20].
- Dietary salt restriction—for Menière disease.
- Diuretics—Menière disease:
  - thiazide diuretics
  - potassium-sparing agents = spironolactone, thiazide + amiloride; at least 3 months of diuretic therapy recommended before discontinuing
    a. sulfa allergies—can try loop diuretics or alternate therapies

- carbon anhydrase inhibitors (acetazolamide)
  a. "inner ear glaucoma"
  b. decreased Na-H exchange in tubule
  c. decreased CSF production
  d. diuretic effects not as long-lasting
  e. dide effects—nephrocalcinosis, mild metabolic acidosis, GI disturbances

- Betahistine (H1-agonist and H3-antagonist)
  - for Menière disease—at least 48 mg tid for at least 6–12 months
  - for unilateral vestibular loss (UVL), to facilitate and enhance vestibular central compensation—48 mg tid for 3 months
  - for bilateral vestibular loss (in the first 3 months)—48 mg tid for 3 months
  - it improves the labyrinthine microcirculation by acting on the precapillary sphincters of the stria vascularis [21] and it reduces the production and increases the absorption of endolymph
- transtympanically gentamicin—20–40 mg/injection at intervals of 4–8 weeks, depending on the efficacy or single-shot injection with follow-up, to avoid ototoxicity for disabling vertigo, after trial of adequate medical therapy [22]. Gentamicin is primarily vestibulotoxic—may impair vestibular dark cells (endolymph), but has an inherent hearing loss risk (30%).
  - gentamicin is injected over round window, with patient supine, ear up for 30 min
  - patients is instructed not to swallow
- low dose of carbamazepine (200–600 mg/day) or oxcarbazepine (300–900 mg/day) for vestibular paroxysmia [23]
  - if these are not tolerated, we can try phenytoin, valproic acid or acetazolamide
- antibiotics, in labyrinthitis and otosyphilis; otosyphilis is treated with the same protocol as neurosyphilis, with Penicillin, if no allergy is present.
  - Intravenous Crystallin Penicillin G 18–24,000,000 UI at 4 h intervals for 10–21 days, continued with intramuscular benzathine Penicillin 2,400,000 UI three times in 1 week.

2.2 Repositioning maneuvers

For benign paroxysmal positional vertigo (BPPV), the most common cause of peripheral vestibular syndrome, treatment is based on physical maneuvers of repositioning the otoconial fragments from the semicircular canal into the utricle.

Canal repositioning procedures differ for each semicircular canal and also for different pathophysiological mechanisms—canalithiasis or cupulolithiasis. For this reason, a precise diagnosis is mandatory, to establish which ear and which semicircular canal is affected, which semicircular canal/ear is affected more in cases of multicanal BPPV and if the otoconial fragments float free or are attached to the cupula.

For diagnostic and treatment as well, there are some contraindications:

- absolute contraindications: cervical spine trauma or recent surgery
- relative contraindications: glaucoma, morbid overweight

For patients with cupulolithiasis, we first try to dislocate the otoconial fragments from the cupula by vibrations applied on the affected mastoid or head-shaking maneuver and transform the cupulolithiasis into a canalithiasis, which has much higher success rate by repositioning treatment.

For patients in whom an appropriate canal repositioning procedure (CRP) is not possible, Brandt–Daroff vestibular habituation exercises are recommended. Otherwise, several CRP is used.

a. canalithiasis of the posterior semicircular canal (pc)—the most frequent affected:

- Semont liberatory maneuver (**Figure 1**): From a sitting position, patient is swiftly placed laterally on the affected ear, with nose facing upwards (i.e., for left posterior semicircular canal canalithiasis, head is turned 45° to the healthy right ear and patient is placed laterally on the left side of the trunk). After nystagmus ceases, the patient is moved quickly through 180° while maintaining the original head position to lie face down on the opposite side. This may trigger further nystagmus and symptoms. Return the patient to the seated position when nystagmus and symptoms stop.

- recently, a variant (Semont plus), is recommended, with better results [24, 25]. The difference from the original Semont maneuver is that in the first position, head is extended off the examination coach.

- Epley canal repositioning procedure (**Figure 2**), with very high rates of success: The patient is seated upright. Turn his head 30–45° to the affected ear. Supporting his head, lie him backward quickly, with the neck slightly hyperextended off the bed. After the nystagmus ceases, turn the patient's head 90° toward the healthy ear. After 2 min in this position, the patient should rotate his body on the healthy side, facilitating further head rotation to 90° (nose towards the ground). This may trigger further nystagmus and symptoms. When the nystagmus and symptoms stop, return the patient to the seated position and bent the head forward for another 2 min.

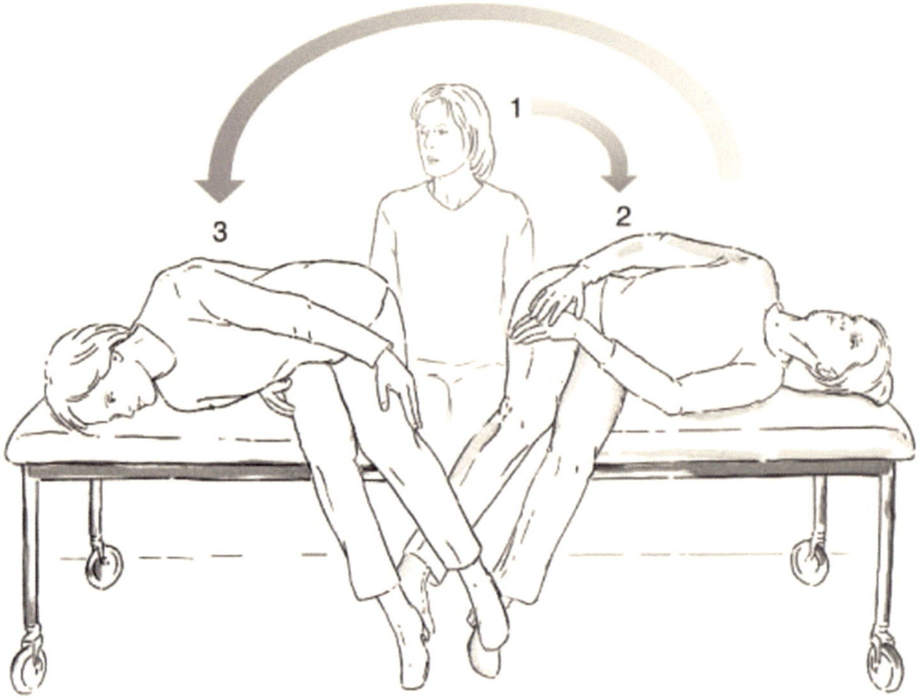

Figure 1.
Semont liberatory maneuver.

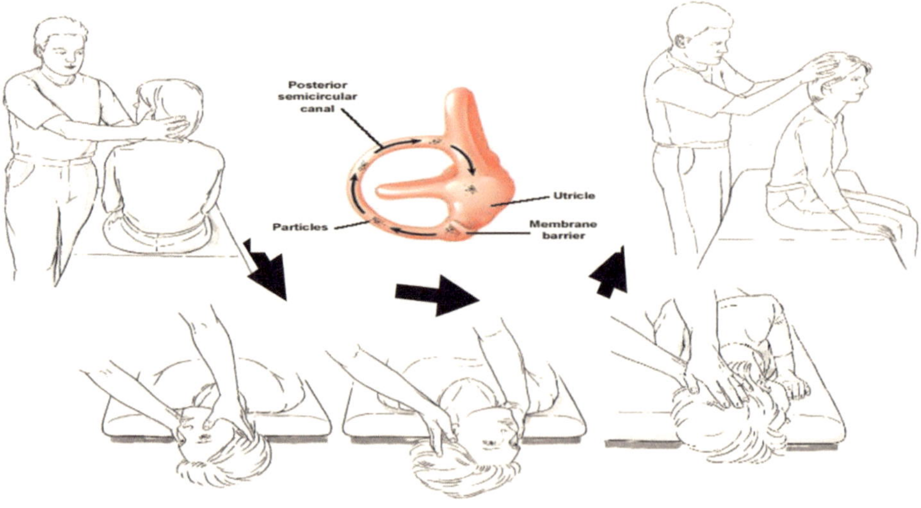

Figure 2.
Epley canalar repositioning maneuver.

b. canalithiasis of the horizontal semicircular canal (hc)—several methods of treatment are used, with variable success rates

- forced prolonged positioning on the healthy side (head and whole body), for 12 h [26]

- "barbecue" maneuver [27] (**Figure 3**). From supine position, patient is turned in steps of 90° toward the healthy ear until laying on the affected ear lateral decubitus and then returned to the sitting position. Each position must be maintained for 1 min.

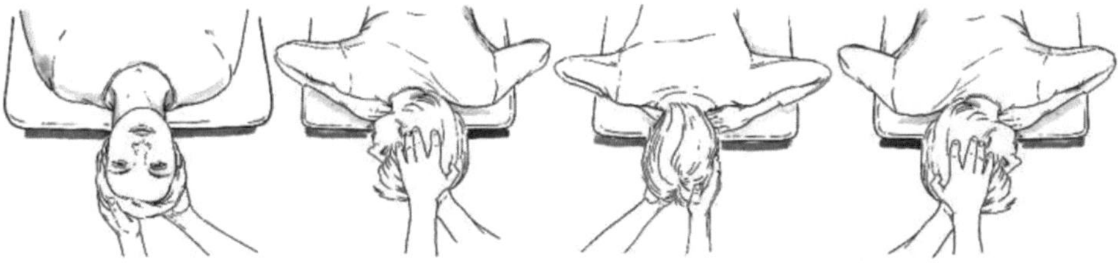

Figure 3.
Barbeque maneuver.

- Gufoni maneuver (**Figure 4**) removes detritus from the horizontal semicircular canal. From the sitting position, patient is brought to the side position on the healthy. After 20 s, the head is rotated in the yaw plane 45° down. After 1–2 min in this position, the patient is brought back to the sitting position, in which the head may rotate back to the neutral position.

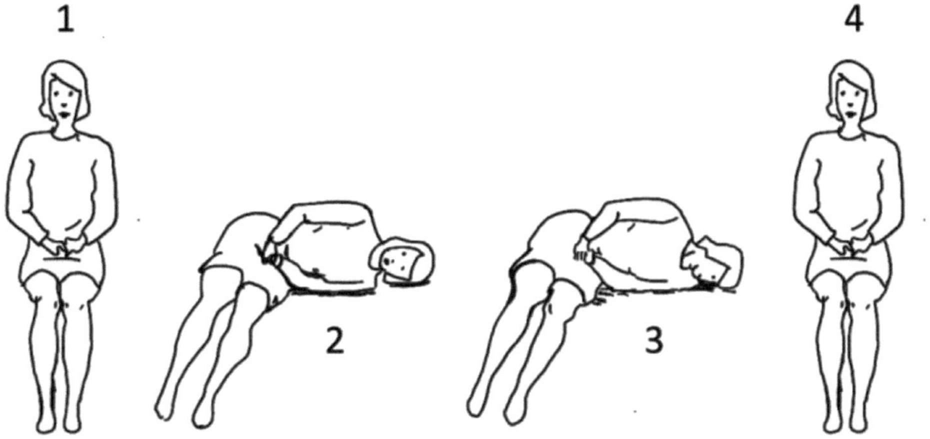

Figure 4.
Gufoni maneuver for right-hc canalithiasis.

c. cupulolithiasis oh the horizontal semicircular canal (hc)—the aim of the liberatory maneuvres is to transform the cupulolithiasis into a canalithiasis, either by modifying the canalithiasis maneuvers, either by applying a vibrator on the affected mastoid during the repositioning maneuver

- Gufoni maneuver (**Figure 5**)—from the sitting position, patient goes to the side position on the affected ear and after 20 s, head is turned for 45° with nose up. After 1–2 min in this position, the patient is brought back to the sitting position, in which the head may rotate back to the neutral position.

- Kim maneuver [28]. From the supine position, patient turns on the affected side and head is turned another 45° towards the lesion side.

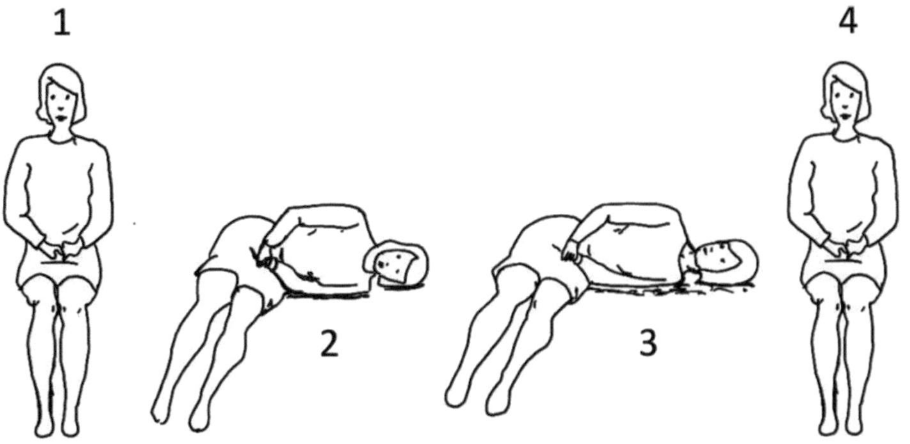

Figure 5.
Gufoni maneuver for left-hc cupulolithiasis.

Vibration is applied on the affected mastoid and then head is turned back 45° towards the healthy ear. In complete lateral decubitus on the affected ear of the patient. Next position of the patient is supine again, followed by lateral decubitus on the healthy side, when vibration is again applied on the healthy ear (for the variant of cupulolithiasis when fragments are on the short arm of the horizontal semicircular canal). Then patient reaches the prone position and slowly the patient is brought back to sitting position without neck extension.

- Zuma maneuver [29]. From the sitting position, patient is swiftly placed on the affected side (upper trunk). After 3 min, head turned upwards 90° and maintained in this position for another 3 min. Next, patient turns into the supine position with the whole body and head is turned 90° towards the healthy ear. After another 3 min, head is tilted forward, and patient returns to the initial position (sitting)

d. anterior semicircular canal (ac) canalithiasis—the rarest form of BPPV, probably because repositioning is taking place spontaneous during night, raised many controverses regarding treatment.

- One of the first treatment options was to perform an Epley maneuver for the healthy ear, taken into consideration the co-planarity of the two vertical semicircular canals—the anterior from one ear and the posterior from the opposite ear, but it proves a low efficiency [30–32].

- The Yacovino maneuver was seen to be an effective treatment option for ac-BPPV without having to determine the side involved. However, simulations showed that the classical Yacovino maneuver carried a risk of canal switch to the posterior canal. The Yacovino maneuver consists of four steps each performed at an interval of 30 s: from the sitting position, patient lies down with head in head-hanging position, 30° below the horizontal plane. After 30 s, head is elevated so that the chin touches the chest and then patient returns to the sitting position [33, 34].

- To overcome this risk, a modified Yacovino maneuver is suggested [35]. In this variation, the subject is brought directly from the head-hanging position to the sitting position. After an interval of 30 s, the neck of the subject is flexed forward at an angle of 45°.

2.3 Vestibular rehabilitation

For stable, definite unilateral vestibula loss (UVL), treatment is more complex because recovery of the long-term deficits induced by UVL should start as soon as possible. As mentioned before, there is a critical period in which the neuroplasticity mechanisms (central vestibular compensation) should start and act at their maximal potential in order to give patients the best opportunities to recover their balance functionality, to return to their daily activities, job, and physical hobbies.

In order to achieve these,

- Symptomatic medical treatment of the acute phase should not exceed 3 days.

- Central compensation process should be facilitated and enhanced by long-term (3 months) treatment with Betahistine and vestibular rehabilitation (VR) customized program [36, 37].

VR promotes vestibular compensation by:

- Habituation mechanisms

- Enhancing adaptation of VOR & VSR

- Substitution strategy of balance (pursuit, saccades)

Physical exercises based treatment, which gradually and progressively stimulates the vestibular system and facilitates vestibular compensation. Starting point is the minimal skill level the patient if able to perform and, as compensation and habituation occurs, speed and complexity of the exercises are increased. Vestibular rehabilitation uses neuroplasticity central mechanisms (adaptation, habituation, sensorial, and functional substitution) to increase static and dynamic postural stability and to improve visual-vestibular interactions [36, 38, 39].

Before vestibular rehabilitation program is designed, a detailed evaluation of equilibrium abilities must be performed, in terms of functionality (gait with head movement, static and dynamic balance in fixed and altered inputs—Timed Up and Go Test, posturography), alternative sensorial systems capabilities (visual and somatosensorial) and fall risk (Unipedal Stance Test).

Also, specific activities and head or body positions that provoke symptoms should be determined.

Today vestibular rehabilitation programs are still based on Cawthorne–Cooksey exercises developed [40] and modified by Susan Herdman [41], due to their excellent results in building up the tolerance. These exercises include eye and head movements, coordination of eyes and head movements (visual-vestibular interaction), postural control exercises, balance tasks with gradually increased difficulty (eyes opened, eyes closed, large base support, uneven base support, while walking, in heavy visual or noisy environments). Exercises are recommended to be performed twice a day, for 30 min, with 10 repetitions of each exercise.

2.3.1 Cawthorne-Cooksey exercises

A. In bed

1. Eye movements: at first slow, then quick
    - up and down
    - from side to side
    - focus on finger while moving from 1 m to 30 cm away from face
2. Head movements: at first slow, then quick. Later with eyes closed.

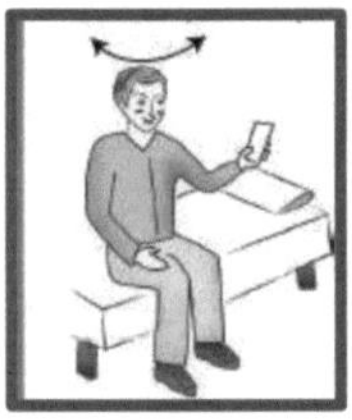

- turn from side to side, shoulder to shoulder
- bend backward and forward

B. Sitting

1 and 2 as above

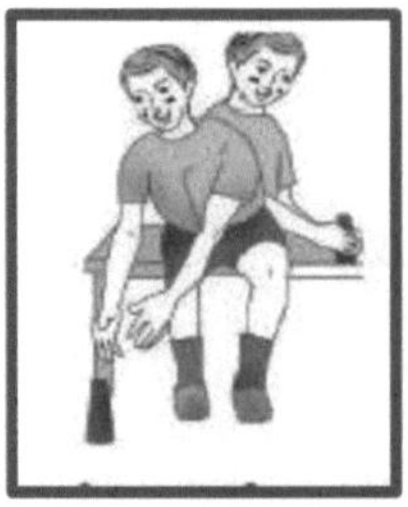

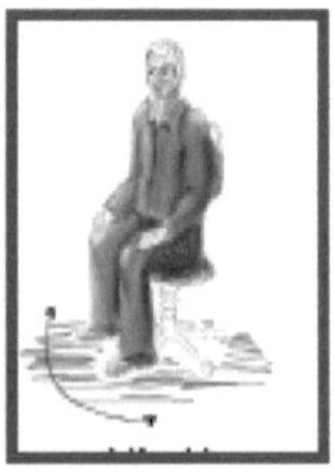

1. Shoulder shrugging and circling
2. Bend forward and pick objects from the ground
3. Rotate on a chair from one side to another, while fixation an image

C. Standing and walking

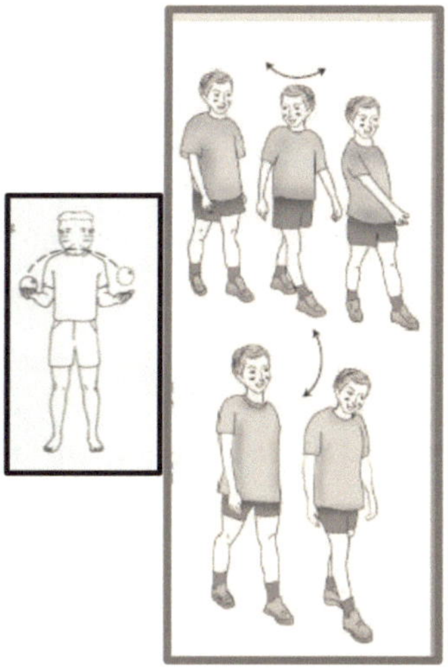

1. As A1, A2 and B3

2. Change from sitting to standing with eyes open, then eyes closed

3. Throw a small ball from hand to hand (above eye level)

4. Throw a ball from hand to hand under the knee

5. Change from sitting to standing and turn around in between

6. Walk 5–7 m distance while moving head side to side, backwards to forwards and from one shoulder to another

2.3.2 Vestibular rehabilitation exercises

At-home exercises are associated, when possible, with weekly sessions of vestibular rehabilitation exercises based on visual feedback (**Figure 6**) on specific equipment, very expensive, unfortunately—Equitest, Bertec, Virtualis, CAREN, etc.

When patients have multifactorial causes of balance difficulty (e.g., elderly with vision disturbances—cataract, peripheral neuropathy, osteoarthritic pathology),

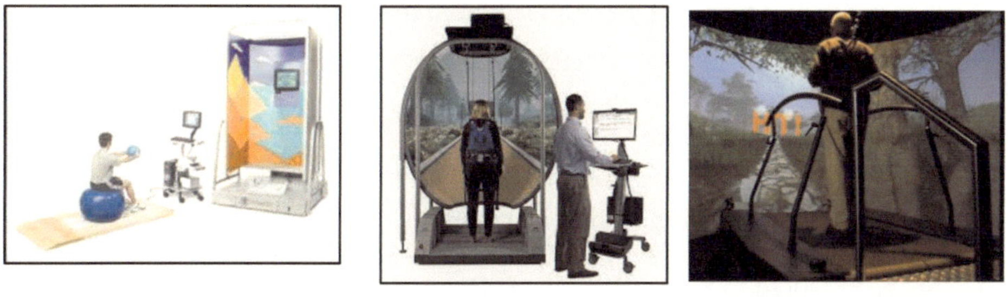

Figure 6
Visual feedback-based vestibular rehabilitation. (a) Equitest-Neurcom. (b) Bertec system. (c) CAREN system.

balance recovery is more difficult and good outcome comes with longer time, but with a positive impact on possible complications of falls. Positive effects on walking, postural control, balance, and mobility in the elderly have been reported with exercises in the form of interactive games where virtual reality technologies are used [42–46].

Vestibular rehabilitation programs must take into consideration some very important factors:

- age (mobility decreases with age)
- patient's daily activity and physical condition—non-sports people versus sportive people
- other comorbidities involve the other sensorial systems involved in balance, vision, proprioception, superficial somatosensorial inputs—tactile receptors (touch, foot pressure) and proprioceptive or deep somatosensory inputs—muscle and tendon stretch receptors. For these patients' safety has to be enforced for at-home exercises, in order to prevent falls.
- for patients with bilateral vestibular loss, VR is the only efficient method in diminishing the severity of gait disturbances. Results come later (after at least 6 months) and treatment lasts for at least 1 year, but usually, some daily exercises are recommended "forever".
- during the COVID-19 pandemic, vestibular rehabilitation was based mainly on telemedicine, with periodic follow-up via internet-based audio and video connection (WhatsApp was affordable for the majority of patients). Hand out and links to instruction films for at-home use were created, available on different websites or especially designed apps. Patient alone is prone to non-adherence and attrition, so he needs ON-LINE support in this HYBRID program. IDEAL—family member available = for patient's SAFETY, especially for:
    - standing and walking exercises in cases of bilateral vestibular loss
    - Epley maneuvre—"Tumarkin-like" attack might appear at the end of the maneuver

These telemedicine solutions are not reimbursed in many countries, and this was a problem for health care providers and patients as well.

There are also some limitations of VR through telemedicine:

- Unstable internet connection
- Type of mobile phone (it has to have a mobile camera and access to the internet)
- Low technology knowledge from the patient
- Hearing impaired patient
- Light intensity in the room

- Correct positioning of the video camera, especially for repositioning maneuvers and walking exercises

Informing and counseling are crucial for coping and therapy adherence. We must explain to the patients the symptoms and inform them explicitly about the impact of and need for treatment. Do not forget that therapy adherence in almost any chronic disease = only 30–50%!!!

For better adherence and compliance of patients to this physical treatment, virtual reality programs are used more and more often, most easily based on Wii and Kinect platforms or virtual reality Googles.

Recent studies demonstrated better results with virtual reality in patients with unilateral peripheral vestibular loss and in elderly. This induces retinal slip and secondary optokinetic eye movements, which stimulate adaptation and compensation mechanisms [47, 48]. Using smartphones for delivering the virtual reality environment proved to be a valid training stimulus, which induces difficulties in postural stability control. Additionally, if a head-mounted system is used, there is a potential to reduce the VOR gain through adaptative changes in the central structures of the vestibular system [49, 50].

Benefit's evaluation of the vestibular rehabilitation.

Physical treatment through vestibular rehabilitation has proven to be a very important instrument in recovery of the vestibular deficit. The benefit has to take into consideration both patient's evaluation as well as health care provider's point of view.

- Subjective evaluation of the UVL-induced handicap and treatment's benefit includes self-evaluation questionnaires:
    - VAS—visual analog scale for symptoms associated with vestibular impairment
    - DHI—Dizziness Handicap Inventory, used for quantification of the severity of the lesion (**Table 1**) and also for treatment's result (improvement with more than 18 points is considered a statistically significant improvement)
    - Activities-specific Balance Confidence (*ABC*) *Scale*
    - Anxiety/depression self-evaluation: HADS-A, HADS-D, because many patients with vestibular impairment experience anxiety, fear, low confidence in their physical independence and even depression
    - Vestibular Rehabilitation Benefit Questionnaire which was recently refined and validated
- Physical performance tests

16–34p	**Mild handicap**
36–52p	Moderate handicap
>54p	Severe handicap

Table 1.
Severity of the vestibular lesion based on DHI score.

- BBS: Berg Balancc Scalc
- SPPB: Short Physical Performance Battery
- POMA: Performance Oriented Mobility Assessment
- DGI: Dynamic Gait Index, very useful for fall risk assessment
- TUG: Timed Up and Go Test

- Clinical vestibular evaluation:
  - for vestibulo-ocular reflex (VOR): presence of nystagmus, head impulse test
  - for vestibulo-spinal reflex (VSR): Romberg test, stepping test, Unipedal Stance Test (excellent predictor for falls)
- Objective vestibular evaluation:
  - CDP: computerized dynamic posturography allows assessment of the vestibulospinal reflex and also visual or proprioception dependence. Recent versions offer additional tests, such as dynamic visual acuity (DVA) and gaze stabilization test (GST)
  - vHIT: video Head Impulse Test
  - cVEMP and oVEMP: cervical and ocular Vestibular Evoked Myogenic Potentials
  - SVV: Subjective Visual Vertical

To summarize, vestibular rehabilitation:

- improves walking, static, and sand dynamic balance
- reduces vestibular symptoms during daily activities
- reduces anxiety and depression induced by AUVL
- increase self-confidence, movement independence, and life quality [51].
- rehab optimizes compensation, sensory substitution, and may lead to new connections and strategies
- but we have to start FAST with rehab (therapeutical window of 8 days after acute loss) for patient's best recovery

Besides unilateral vestibular loss, many patients experience bilateral vestibular hypofunction (such as aging of the vestibular system in elderly = presbivestibulia) or even bilateral vestibular loss (bvl). They struggle to maintain balance, especially when walking in the dark or on uneven surfaces and present oscillopsia during walking or head movements. Central vestibular compensation can not occur in these cases due to bilateral impairment, so patients' recovery is much more difficult, and imperfect. BVL leads up to 30 times higher risk of falling, significant loss of quality of life, and an increased socio-economic burden on individuals and on society [52]. The etiologies of BVL vary from ototoxicity (e.g., aminoglycoside treatment or chemotherapy), to genetic factors (e.g., DFNA9), CANVAS or spinocerebellar ataxia, infectious causes (meningitis), autoimmunity (e.g., Cogan's syndrome), trauma, and neurodegenerative diseases [53–55].

In some patients, there may be a transition from presbyvestibulopathy to BVP due to aging or neurodegeneration [56, 57].

New methods of treatment for bilateral vestibular loss are also available, only in clinical studies for the moment:

2.3.3 Vestibular prothesis: Balance Belt

A wearable (hip belt) medical device which provides haptic feedback to improve balance and mobility in patients with severe bilateral vestibular loss (**Figure 7**) [58]. Patients improved their independent balance, moved without relying on somebody else or walking cane.

The Balance Belt, developed by Professor Herman Kingma, contains several tiny vibration motors and an accelerometer which sense the direction the wearer is leaning toward and provides vibrational feedback to alert the wearer about their self-movement and body position. The wearer interprets the feedback subconsciously, corrects their posture, and improves their balance this way.

According to the inventor: "A sensor in the belt feels, as it were, where gravity is. If someone moves too far in the wrong direction, the belt produces vibrations. This is just enough to make sure you do not get out of balance and gain just a little bit more certainty."

2.3.4 Vestibular implant (VI)

Vestibular implant (VI) (**Figure 8**) is a self-contained system that provides artificial sensation of head rotation by electrically stimulating the three semicircular canal branches of the vestibular nerve [59]. As for cochlear implant, vestibular implant is an

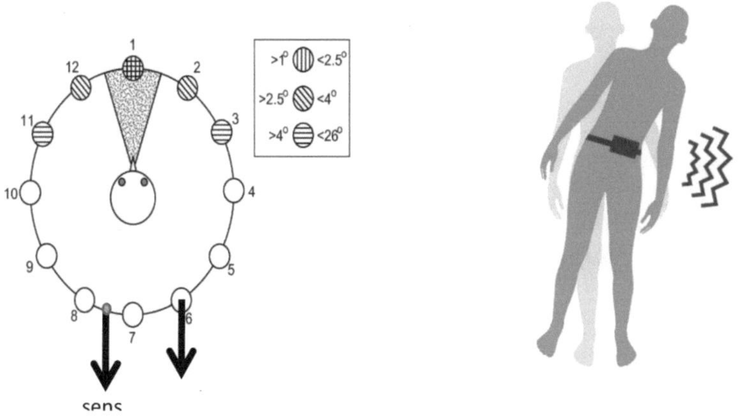

Figure 7.
Balance belt.

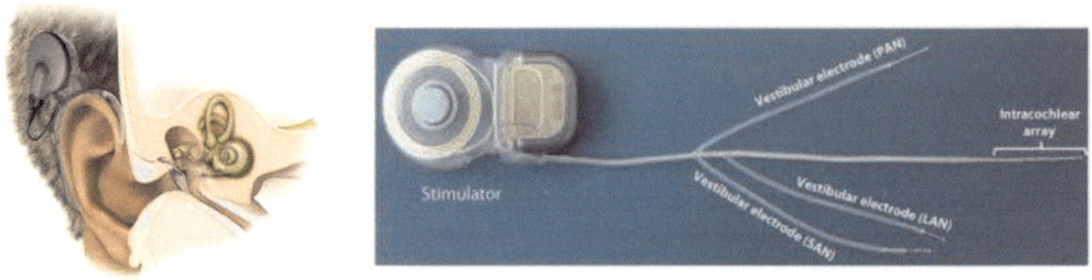

Figure 8.
Vestibular implant (Source: MED EL Company).

artificial replacement of the non-functional vestibular end organ, which captures head movement through motion sensors and sends electrical signals to the vestibular nerves by electrodes that are implanted near the vestibular nerve branches that innervate the semicircular canals and the otolith organs [60–63].

Clinical studies showed an increase in the vestibulo-ocular gain [64–67], an improvement of vestibulospinal and vestibulocollic reflexes [68, 69] and restoration of the dynamic visual acuity in difficult high-frequency head movements [70, 71].

The criteria for VI-implantation should go beyond the existing criteria for BVP, in order to demonstrate significant impairment of all canals in all frequency ranges, and (on indication) the otolith organs, because implantation would destroy residual vestibular function [72].

Criteria for vestibular implant eligibility are:

A. Chronic vestibular impairment with 2 disabling symptoms of unsteadiness when walking or standing plus at least one of the following:

  - Movement-induced blurred vision or oscillopsia during walking or quick head/body movements, and/or

  - Worsening of unsteadiness in darkness and/or on uneven ground

B. Head movement induces the most severe symptoms.

C. Bilaterally reduced or absent angular VOR function documented by at least one of the following major criteria:

  - Bilaterally pathological horizontal angular VOR gain ≤ 0.6 and at least bilaterally one vertical angular VOR gain < 0.7, measured by the video-HIT or scleral-coil technique. Angular eye velocity is measured at a fixed time (around 60 ms after onset of the impulse), minimum of seven artifact-free impulses, with peak acceleration of at least $1000/s^2$ [73]. Only one vertical semicircular canal on each side needs to fulfill the criterion of an angular VOR gain < 0.7, since it was shown that selective sparing of a single semicircular canal is possible [74] while a clinically relevant BVP is still present, making the patient probably eligible for implantation.

  - Reduced caloric response (sum of bithermal max. Peak SPV on each side $\leq 6°/s$ for 30 s water stimuli or $< 10°/s$ for 60 s water or air stimuli). Irrigations of water, lasting for ≥ 30 s, with a total volume of at least 250 ml and 5 min interval between successive irrigations [73]. For air stimulus, 8 l/min for at least 60 s should be used. Patients with a sum of all bithermal irrigations <20°/s still reported significant imbalance and/or oscillopsia [53, 75].

- Reduced horizontal angular VOR gain ≤0.1 upon sinusoidal stimulation on a rotatory chair (0.1 Hz, Vmax = 50°/s) and a phase lead >68° (time constant <5 s).

C′. Obligatory only in case of implantation of otolith structures: Bilaterally absent cVEMP and oVEMP responses.

D. In case only one or two criteria from C are matched (and also criterion C′ is matched in case of otolith stimulation), the remaining test(s) should comply with the following minor criteria:

- Bilaterally pathological VOR gains of at least two semicircular canals <0.7, measured by the video-HIT or scleral-coil technique.
- Reduced caloric response (sum of bithermal max. Peak SPV on each side <10°/s for water and air stimuli of ≥30 s).
- Reduced horizontal angular VOR gain <0.2 upon sinusoidal stimulation on a rotatory chair (0.1 Hz, Vmax = 50°/s).

E. Symptoms are not better accounted for by another disease.

F. Fitting the additional requirements relevant to initial preclinical trials.

- Age 18 years and above.
- BVP results most likely from a peripheral origin [55].
- An improvement in patient's vestibular function is unlikely [76] (6 months "wait-and-see" period).
- Patent vestibular end-organ and intact vestibular nerve [56] and no chronic otitis media.
- Ability to use the device and follow a personalized rehabilitation program.
- Ability to undergo the surgery [57].

G. No current psychological or psychiatric disorder that could significantly interfere with the use or evaluation of the VI [73].

SHIMP test was not included in the evaluation of the vestibular function since the clinical relevance of SHIMPs in BVP should still be determined [77].

Handicap Inventory total score of >30 would be preferred since this could show at least moderate handicap [78–80]. But this is not mandatory if we discuss about eligibility criteria for vestibular implantation.

With absent cVEMP and oVEMP responses, it is expected that the benefit of vestibular implantation will be higher than the drawbacks of the potential iatrogenically induced vestibular hypofunction due to vestibular implantation of the otolith endorgans.

Surgery for vestibular implantation implies inserting the electrodes either in the proximity of the ampullae of the semicircular canals by opening the semicircular canals or the vestibulum (intralabyrinthine approach), either in the vicinity of the vestibular nerve branches on the semicircular canals end or in the internal auditory canal (extralabyrinthine approach) [81]. Each surgical option has its risks—loss of residual hearing for the intralabyrinthine approach and exposure and damage of the facial nerve for the extralabyrinthine approach [82].

Since implantation of otolith structures [60] is almost certain to cause otolith hypofunction due to mechanical disruption of the membranous labyrinth during implantation, oVEMPS and cVEMPS were included in the implantation criteria when the otolith structures will be replaced by the vestibular implant.

3. Conclusion

Peripheral vestibular lesions are found in more than 50% of patients with vestibular impairment. First three etiologies of peripheral vestibular lesions are BPPV, vestibular neuritis and Menière's disease, each of them with specific treatment management, different in between.

Only this is solid argument for continuously updating our knowledge in the field, in order to offer best treatment option to our patients—appropriate repositioning maneuver, acute or subacute and chronic medical treatment or vestibular rehabilitation individualized programs.

Vestibular impairment, most frequently unilateral, decrease mobility, equilibrium and impair patient's daily activities and his job skills, with a decreased overall quality of life.

Some vestibular disorders have a negative impact upon patient's daily mental status, like Menière's disease with its unpredictable acute attacks. Others, like vestibular neuritis patients, have a long-lasting functional impairment and imply long-term recovery treatment (medical and physical) which will facilitate and enhance the natural recovery mechanism of central vestibular compensation.

Bilateral vestibular hypofunction (e.g., elderly) or bilateral vestibular loss is much more difficult to treat, because vestibular neuroplasticity does not work in these cases. For these patients, specific vestibular rehabilitation programs were designed, more recently with specific virtual reality exercises included for better adherence and compliance to years of rehabilitation.

Also, as research studies for the moment, specific medical devices were designed—vibrotactile Balance Belt and vestibular implant.

Conflict of interest

The author declares no conflict of interest.

DOI: http://dx.doi.org/10.5772/intechopen.107103

Author details

Madalina Georgescu
Audiology and Clinical Hearing Aid Department, "Carol Davila" University of Medicine and Pharmacy, Bucharest, Romania

*Address all correspondence to: madalina.georgescu@gecad.com

References

[1] Neuhauser HK. Epidemiology of vertigo. Current Opinion in Neurology. 2007;**20**:40-46

[2] Grill E, Heuberger M, Strobl R, et al. Prevalence, determinants, and consequences of vestibular hypofunction. Results from the KORA-FF4 survey. Frontiers in Neurology. 2018;**9**:1076

[3] Agrawal Y, Carey JP, Della Santina CC, Schubert MC, Minor LB. Disorders of balance and vestibular function in US adults: Data from the National Health and Nutrition Examination Survey, 2001–2004. Archives of Internal Medicine. 2009 May 25;**169**(10):938-944

[4] Huppert D, Strupp M, Muckter H, Brandt T. Which medication do I need to manage dizzy patients? Acta Oto-Laryngologica. 2011;**131**:228-241

[5] Lacour M, Sterkers O. Histamine and betahistine in the treatment of vertigo: Elucidation of mechanisms of action. CNS Drugs. 2001;**15**:853-870

[6] Hillier SL, Hollohan V. Vestibular rehabilitation for unilateral peripheral vestibular dysfunction. Cochrane Database of Systematic Reviews. 2007; **17**:CD005397

[7] Kammerlind AS, Ledin TE, Odkvist LM, Skargren EI. Effects of home training and additional physical therapy on recovery after acute unilateral vestibular loss-a randomized study. Clinical Rehabilitation. 2005;**19**: 54-62

[8] Shepard NT, Telian SA, Smith-Wheelock M, Raj A. Vestibular and balance rehabilitation therapy. The Annals of Otology, Rhinology, and Laryngology. 1993;**102**:198-205

[9] Georgescu M. Vestibular rehabilitation – Recommended treatment for permanent unilateral vestibular loss. International Journal of Neurorehabilitation. 2017;**4**:282. DOI: 10.4172/2376-0281.1000282

[10] Hall CD, Herdman SJ, Whitney SL, Cass SP, Clendaniel RA, et al. Vestibular rehabilitation for peripheral vestibular hypofunction: An evidence-based clinical practice guideline. Journal of Neurologic Physical Therapy. 2016;**40**:124-155. DOI: 10.1097/NPT.0000000000000120 PMID: 26913496

[11] Georgescu M, Sorina S. Vestibular neuronitis in pregnancy. GINECO eu. 2011;7:58-61

[12] Madalina G, Sorina S, Aurelia MC, Gh.V C. Vestibulary rehabilitation – election treatment method for compensating vestibular impairment. Romanian Journal of Morphology and Embryology. 2012;**53**(3):651-656

[13] Georgescu M. Vestibular rehabilitation – recommended treatment for permanent unilateral vestibular loss. International Journal of Neurorehabilitation. 2017;**4**:4. DOI: 10.4172/2376-0281.1000282

[14] Georgescu M. Central vestibular compensation. Canadian Hearing Report. Revue Canadienne d' audition. 2018;**13**(1):7-11 Andrew John Publishing

[15] Herdman SJ. Vestibular Rehabilitation. 4th ed. 2014. p. 597

[16] Smith PF, Darlington CL, Curthoys IS. Vestibular compensation without brainstem commissures in the

guinea pig. Neuroscience Letters. 1986; **65**:209-221. DOI: 10.1016/0304-3940 (86)90306-x PMID: 3487051

[17] Smith PF, Darlington CL, Curthoys IS. The effect of visual deprivation in vestibular compensation in the guinea pig. Brain Research. 1986; **364**:195-198. DOI: 10.1016/0006-8993 (86)91004-8

[18] Zee DS. Vestibular adaptation In: Herdman S, editor. Vestibular Rehabilitation. 3rd ed. F.A. Davis: F. A. Company; 2007. pp. 19-31

[19] Gurley JM, Hujsak BD, Kelly JL. Vestibular rehabilitation following mild traumatic brain injury. NeuroRehabilitation. 2013;**32**(3):519-528

[20] Strupp M, Zingler VC, Arbusow V, et al. Methylprednisolone, valacyclovir, or the combination for vestibular neuritis. The New England Journal of Medicine. 2004;**351**:354-361

[21] Yilmaz I, Yilmazer C, Erkan AN, Aslan SG, Ozluoglu LN. Intratympanic dexamethasone injection effects on transient-evoked otoacoustic emission. American Journal of Otolaryngology. 2005;**26**:113-117

[22] Dziadziola JK, Laurikainen EL, Rachel JD, Quirk WS. Betahistine increases vestibular blood flow. Otolaryngology and Head and Neck Surgery. 1999;**120**:400-405

[23] Lange G, Maurer J, Mann W. Long-term results after interval therapy with intratympanic gentamicin for Meniere's disease. Laryngoscope. 2004;**114**: 102-105

[24] Hufner K, Barresi D, Glaser M, et al. Vestibular paroxysmia: Diagnostic features and medical treatment. Neurology. 2008;**71**:1006-1014

[25] Michael Strupp, Nicolina Goldschagg, Anne-Sophie Vinck, Otmar Bayer, Sebastian Vandenbroeck, Lorenzo Salerni, Anita Hennig, Dominik Obrist, Marco Mandalà. BPPV: Comparison of the SémontPLUS with the Sémont maneuver: A prospective randomized trial. Neurology. 14 Apr 2021;**12**:662573. DOI: 10.3389/fneur.2021.652573

[26] Anita Bhandari, Rajneesh Bhandari, Herman Kingma, Michael Strupp. Diagnostic and Therapeutic Maneuvers for Anterior Canal BPPV Canalithiasis: Three-Dimensional Simulations. E-Collection 24 Sep 2021;**12**:740599. DOI: 10.3389/fneur.2021.740599

[27] Vannucchi P, Pagnini P, Giannoni B, et al. Terapia fisica dela vPPB del cSO: Posizione liberatoria coatta. In: Motta G, editor. Atti del LXXXI Congresso Nazionale della Societa' Italiana di Otorinolaringoiatriae Chirurgia Cervico Facciale. Pisa: Pacini; 1994. p. 179

[28] Lempert T. Horizontal benign positional vertigo. Neurology. 1994;**44**: 2213-2214

[29] Kim SH, Jo SW, Chung WK, et al. A cupulolith repositioning maneuver in the treatment of horizontal canal cupulolithiasis. Auris Nasus Larynx. 2012;**39**:163-168

[30] Zuma e Maia F. New treatment strategy for apogeotropic horizontal canal benign paroxysmal positional vertigo. Audiology Research. 2016;**6**:163

[31] Honrubia V, Baloh RW, Harris MR, Jacobson KM. Paroxysmal positional vertigo syndrome. The American Journal of Otology. 1999;**20**:465-470

[32] Epley JM. Human experience with canaliths repositioning maneuvers. Annals of the New York Academy of

Sciences. 2001;**942**:179-191. DOI: 10.1111/j.1749-6632.2001.tb03744.x

[33] Seok J, Lee H, Yoo J, Lee D. Residual dizziness after successful repositioning treatment in patients with benign paroxysmal positional vertigo. Journal of Clinical Neurology. 2008;**4**:107. DOI: 10.3988/jcn.2008.4.3.107

[34] Hain TC, Squires TM, Stone HA. Clinical implications of a mathematical model of benign paroxysmal positional vertigo. Annals of the New York Academy of Sciences. 2005;**1039**: 384-394. DOI: 10.1196/annals.1325.036

[35] Eggers SDZ, Zee DS. Vertigo and Imbalance: Clinical Neurophysiology of the Vestibular System. Amsterdam: Elsevier; 2010. p. xx

[36] Crane BT, Schessel DA, Nedzelski J, Minor LB. Peripheral vestibular disorders. In: Flint PW, Haughey BH, Lund VJ, et al., editors. Cummings Otolaryngology: Head and Neck Surgery. 5th ed. Philadelphia, PA, USA: Mosby Elsevier; 2010. pp. 2328-2345

[37] Bamiou DE, Luxon LM. Vertigo: Clinical management and rehabilitation. In: Gleeson M, Luxon LM, editors. Scott-Brown's Otorhinolaryngology, Head and Neck Surgery. 7th ed. New York, NY, USA: CRC Press; 2008. pp. 3791-3817

[38] Yacovino D, Hain T, Gualtieri F. New therapeutic maneuver for anterior canal benign paroxysmal positional vertigo. Journal of Neurology. 2009;**256**: 1851-1855. DOI: 10.1007/s00415-009-5208-1

[39] Curthoys IS, Halmagyi GM. Vestibular compensation. In: Buttner U, editor. Vestibular Dysfunction and its Therapy. Advances in Otorhinolaryngology. Basel, Switzerland: Karger; 1999. pp. 195-227

[40] Gans RE. Vestibular rehabilitation: Critical decision analysis. Seminars in Hearing. 2002;**23**(2):149-159

[41] Cawthorne T. The physiological basis for head exercises. The Chartered Society of Physiotherapy. 1944;**30**: 106-107

[42] Duque G, Boersma D, Loza-Diaz G, Hassan S, Suarez H, Geisinger D, et al. Effects of balance training using a virtual-reality systemin older fallers. Clinical Interventions in Aging. 2013;**8**: 257-263

[43] Toulotte C, Toursel C, Olivier N. Wii Fit(R) training vs. adapted physical activities: Which one is the most appropriate to improve the balance of independent senior subjects? A randomized controlled study. Clinical Rehabilitation. 2012;**26**:827-835

[44] Pichierri G, Murer K, De Bruin ED. A cognitive-motor inter-vention using a dance video game to enhance foot placementaccuracy and gait under dual task conditions in older adults: A randomized controlled trial. BMC Geriatrics. 2012;**12**:74

[45] Laver K, George S, Ratcliffe J, Quinn S, Whitehead C, Davies O, et al. Use of an interactive video gaming program comparedwith conventional physiotherapy for hospitalised older adults: A feasibility trial. Disability and Rehabilitation 2012;**34**:1802–1808

[46] Szturm T, Betker AL, Moussavi Z, Desai A, Goodman V. Effectsof an interactive computer game exercise regimen on balanceimpairment in frail community-dwelling older adults: A randomized controlled trial. Physical Therapy. 2011;**91**:1449-1462

[47] Hall CD, Meldrum D, Whitney SL. The role of emerging technologies in vestibular rehabilitation. In: Herdman SJ, Clendenial RA, editors. Vestibular Rehabilitation. 4th ed. Philadelphia: FA Davis Company; 2014. pp. 537-553

[48] Alrwaily M, Whitney SL. Older adults with dizziness: Rehabilitation strategies and novel interventions. In: Kesser BW, Gleason AT, editors. Dizziness and Vertigo Across the Lifespan. Vol. 44. No. 2. Elsevier Health Sciences; 2011. pp. 473-496

[49] Rausch M, Simon JE, Starkey C, Grooms DR. Smartphone virtualreality to increase clinical balance assessment responsiveness. Physical Therapy in Sport. 2018;**32**:207-211

[50] Di Girolamo S, Picciotti P, Sergi B, Di Nardo W, Paludetti G, Ottaviani F. Vestibulo-ocular reflex modification after virtua lenvironment exposure. Acta Oto-Laryngologica. 2000;**121**:211-215

[51] Ricci NA, Aratani MC, Don'a F, Macedo C, Caovilla HH, Gananca FF. A systematic review about the effects of the vestibular rehabilitation in middle-age and older adults. Revista Brasileira de Fisioterapia. 2010;**14**(5):361-371

[52] Sun DQ, Ward BK, Semenov YR, Carey JP, Santina CCD. Bilateral vestibular deficiency: Quality of life and economic implications. JAMA Otolaryngology. Head & Neck Surgery. Jun 2014;**140**(6):527-534

[53] Lucieer F, Vonk P, Guinand N, Stokroos R, Kingma H, van de Berg R. Bilateral vestibular hypofunction: Insights in etiologies, clinical subtypes, and diagnostics. Frontiers in Neurology. 2016;7:26

[54] Szmulewicz DJ, McLean CA, MacDougall HG, Roberts L, Storey E, Halmagyi GM. CANVAS an update: Clinical presentation, investigation and management. Journal of Vestibular Research: Equilibrium & Orientation. 2014;**24**(5–6):465-474

[55] de Varebeke SP, Termote B, Van Camp G, Govaerts PJ, Schepers S, Cox T, et al. Focal sclerosis of semicircular canals with severe DFNA9 hearing impairment caused by a P51S COCH-mutation: Is there a link? Otology & Neurotology. 2014;**35**(6):1077-1086

[56] Agrawal Y, Van de Berg R, Wuyts F, Walther L, Magnusson M, Oh E, et al. Presbyvestibulopathy: Diagnostic criteria Consensus document of the classification committee of the Barany Society. Journal of Vestibular Research: Equilibrium & Orientation. 2019;**29**(4): 161-170

[57] Miffon M, Guyot JP. Difficulties faced by patients suffering from total bilateral vestibular loss. ORL: Journal for Otorhinolaryngology and Its Related Specialties. 2015;**77**(4):241-247

[58] Herman Kingma, Lilian Felipe, Marie-Cecile Gerards, Peter Gerits, Nils Guinand, Angelica Perez-Fornos, Vladimir Demkin, Raymond van de Berg. Vibrotactile feedback improves balance and mobility in patients with severe bilateral vestibular loss. Journal of Neurology 2019;**266** (Suppl.1):S19–S26. https://doi.org/10.1007/s00415-018-9133-z

[59] Chow MR, Ayiotis AI, Schoo DP, Gimmon Y, Lane KE, Morris BJ, et al. Posture, gait, quality of life, and hearing with a vestibular implant. The New England Journal of Medicine. 2021;**384**: 521-532

[60] Ramos de Miguel A, Falcon Gonzalez JC, Ramos Macias A. Vestibular response to electrical stimulation of the otolith organs. implications in the development of a vestibular implant for

the improvement of the sensation of gravitoinertial accelerations. The Journal of International Advanced Otology. 2017; **13**(2):154-161

[61] Fridman GY, Della Santina CC. Progress toward development of a multichannel vestibular prosthesis for treatment of bilateral vestibular deficiency. Anatomical Record. 2012; **295**(11):2010-2029

[62] Rubinstein JT, Bierer S, Kaneko C, Ling L, Nie K, Oxford T, et al. Implantation of the semicircular canals with preservation of hearing and rotational sensitivity: A vestibular neurostimulator suitable for clinical research. Otology & Neurotology. 2012; **33**(5):789-796

[63] van de Berg R, Guinand N, Ranieri M, Cavuscens S, Khoa Nguyen TA, Guyot JP, et al. The vestibular implant input interacts with residual natural function. Frontiers in Neurology. 2017;**8**:644

[64] Phillips C, Ling L, Oxford T, Nowack A, Nie K, Rubinstein JT, et al. Longitudinal performance of an implantable vestibular prosthesis. Hearing Research. 2015;**322**: 200-211

[65] van de Berg R, Guinand N, Nguyen TA, Ranieri M, Cavuscens S, Guyot JP, et al. The vestibular implant: Frequency-dependency of the electrically evoked vestibulocular reflex in humans. Frontiers in Systems Neuroscience. 2014;**8**:255

[66] Boutros PJ, Schoo DP, Rahman M, Valentin NS, Chow MR, Ayiotis AL, et al. Continuous vestibular implant stimulation partially restores eye-stabilizing reflexes. Journal of Clinical Investigation Insight. 14 Nov 2019;**4**(22)

[67] Rubinstein JT, Ling L, Nowack A, Nie K, Phillips JO. Results from a second-generation vestibular implant in human subjects: Diagnosis may impact electrical sensitivity of vestibular afferents. Otology & Neurotology. 2020;**41**(1):68-77

[68] Fornos AP, van de Berg R, Armand S, Cavuscens S, Ranieri M, Cretallaz C, et al. Cervical myogenic potentials and controlled postural responses elicited by a prototype vestibular implant. Journal of Neurology. 2019;**266**(Suppl. 1):33-41

[69] Phillips C, Defrancisci C, Ling L, Nie K, Nowack A, Phillips JO, et al. Postural responses to electrical stimulation of the vestibular end organs in human subjects. Experimental Brain Research. 2013;**229**(2):181-195

[70] Guinand N, Van de Berg R, Cavuscens S, Stokroos R, Ranieri M, Pelizzone M, et al. Restoring visual acuity in dynamic conditions with a vestibular implant. Frontiers in Neuroscience. 2016;**10**:577

[71] Starkov D, Guinand N, Lucieer F, Ranieri M, Cavuscens S, Pleshkov M, et al. Restoring the high-frequency dynamic visual acuity with a vestibular implant prototype in humans. Audiology & Neuro-Otology. 2019:1-5

[72] van de Berg R, Ramos A, van Rompaey V, et al. The vestibular implant: Opinion statement on implantation criteria for research. Journal of Vestibular Research. 2020;**30**: 213-223. DOI: 10.3233/VES-200701

[73] van de Berg R, van Tilburg M, Kingma H. Bilateral vestibular hypofunction: Challenges in establishing the diagnosis in adults. ORL: Journal for Otorhinolaryngology and Its Related Specialties. 2015;**77**(4):197-218

[74] Tarnutzer AA, Bockisch CJ, Buffone E, Weiler S, Bachmann LM, Weber KP. Disease-specific sparing of the anterior semicircular canals in bilateral vestibulopathy. Clinical Neurophysiology. 2016;**127**(8):2791-2801

[75] Kim S, Oh YM, Koo JW, Kim JS. Bilateral vestibulopathy: Clinical characteristics and diagnostic criteria. Otology & Neurotology. 2011;**32**(5): 812-817

[76] Zingler VC, Cnyrim C, Jahn K, Weintz E, Fernbacher J, Frenzel C, et al. Causative factors and epidemiology of bilateral vestibulopathy in 255 patients. Annals of Neurology. 2007;**61**(6): 524-532

[77] MacDougall HG, McGarvie LA, Halmagyi GM, Rogers SJ, Manzari L, Burgess AM, et al. A new saccadic indicator of peripheral vestibular function based on the video head impulse test. Neurology. 2016;**87**(4): 410-418

[78] B. Dobbels, F. Lucieer, G. Mertens, A. Gilles, J. Moyaert, P. van de Heyning, et al. Vestibular Testing and its Relationship to Symptoms and Falls in 119 Patients with Bilateral Vestibulopathy. 32nd Politzer Society Meeting; Warsaw, 2019. R. van de Berg et al. Vestibular implantation criteria 223

[79] Tamber AL, Wilhelmsen KT, Strand LI. Measurement properties of the Dizziness Handicap Inventory by cross-sectional and longitudinal designs. Health and Quality of Life Outcomes. 2009;**7**:101

[80] Whitney SL, Wrisley DM, Brown KE, Furman JM. Is perception of handicap related to functional performance in persons with vestibular dysfunction? Otology & Neurotology. 2004;**25**(2):139-143

[81] van de Berg R, Guinand N, Guyot JP, Kingma H, Stokroos RJ. The modified ampullar approach for vestibular implant surgery: Feasibility and its first application in a human with a long-term vestibular loss. Frontiers in Neurology. 2012;**3**:18

[82] Feigl GC, Fasel JH, Anderhuber F, Ulz H, Rienmuller R, Guyot JP, et al. Superior vestibular neurectomy: A novel transmeatal approach for a denervation of the superior and lateral semicircular canals. Otology & Neurotology. 2009; **30**(5):586-591

Chapter 5

Vestibular Rehabilitation: Conventional and Virtual Reality-Based Methods

Başak Mutlu

Abstract

The vestibular system is responsible for sensing the velocity and acceleration of angular and linear movements of the head and sensitivity to gravity in maintaining balance with its peripheral and central structures. It performs this function through vestibular reflexes. When peripheral vestibular diseases occur unilaterally or bilaterally, the functions of vestibular reflexes are affected, resulting in deterioration in eye movements compatible with head movements and anti-gravity muscle activity coordination, which ensures upright posture against gravity. Dizziness and/or imbalance persist in patients in whom the central compensation process cannot be completed, resulting in restrictions in the patient's independent movements, daily activities, and quality of life. In the middle and long term, these restrictions cause sedentary life, fear of falling, loss of general condition, emotional problems, and social isolation. In patients diagnosed with unilateral peripheral vestibular disease, vestibular rehabilitation methods based on exercise and living environment arrangements are used as valid and reliable methods to support central compensation mechanisms and to eliminate movement restrictions. Along with conventional exercises, virtual reality-based vestibular rehabilitation systems on stable or unstable platforms are also used for this purpose. In this chapter, the essential principles of conventional and virtual reality-based vestibular rehabilitation methods take place.

Keywords: vestibular disorders, imbalance, central compensation, vestibular rehabilitation, virtual reality

1. Introduction

The vestibular nuclear complex integrates and stores inputs from the vestibular, visual, and proprioceptive sensors. With its central and peripheral connections, the vestibular system provides cortical awareness of head and body movements, control of oculomotor activity, control of posture, and control of motor skills. The vestibular system is also known to contribute to high-level cognitive processes, including spatial perception, spatial navigation, body representation, attention, memory, mental imagery, and social cognition. Therefore, in addition to weakening the vestibular reflexes in vestibular disorders, spatial navigation and memory tasks, as well as body representation and body awareness are impaired. The functional, psychological, and social effects of vestibular diseases are very important from a societal perspective [1, 2].

Vestibular sensors are located in the petrous part of the temporal bone in both inner ears, in anatomical and physiological relationship with the cochlea. The outer part is the bone labyrinth, the inner part is the membranous labyrinth. The membranous labyrinth is filled with endolymph. The space between the bony labyrinth and the membranous labyrinth is filled with perilymph. Perilymph is similar to cerebrospinal fluid. Endolymph is similar to intracellular fluid (high $K+$ and low $Na+$). The sensory structures are located in the membranous labyrinth. Sensory receptors in the vestibular organs are located close to the vertical and horizontal planes. In this way, they can detect all movements of the head. All receptors are excited by forces associated with acceleration. The utricle and saccule (otolith organs) are sensitive to linear acceleration, gravity, and head stability. Semicircular canals are sensitive to angular acceleration in their plane. Vestibular sensors differ from other sensory receptors because they produce motor reflexes as well as positional perception. The sensors of the vestibular labyrinth are innervated by the afferent and efferent fibers of the vestibular branch of the eighth cranial nerve. Nerve fibers form the Scarpa's ganglion go to the brain stem as the vestibular nerve. The vestibular nerve divides into superior and inferior branches and contains a total of 18,000 to 20,000 nerve fibers. The superior branch innervates the utricle, the antero-superior part of the saccule, and the superior and horizontal semicircular canals. The inferior vestibular nerve innervates most of the saccule and the inferior semicircular canal. Most of the vestibular nerve terminates in the vestibular nuclei and a small part in the cerebellum. The vestibular nuclei are located in the posterior part of the brainstem where the pontomedullary junction. There are four major nuclei (superior, lateral, medial, and inferior) and seven minor nuclei separately on the right and left sides of the brain stem. In addition to vestibular inputs, the vestibular nuclear complex also receives inputs from the visual, proprioceptive, cerebellar, and reticular formations. Since the cerebellum is the motor coordination center, it plays a role in the regulation of vestibular reflexes. Cerebellum has a predominantly inhibitory effect on the vestibular nuclear complex. Connections between the cerebellum and vestibular nuclei help maintain balance and posture by providing harmony between head, trunk, and eye movements. Inputs from vestibular sensors are used to create vestibular reflexes that help maintain balance. Vestibular reflexes (vestibulo-ocular, vestibulo-spinal, vestibulo-collic, cervico-ocular, and cervico-collic reflexes) are reflexes that play a role in maintaining balance as a result of processing the visual, proprioceptive, and vestibular inputs at the level of the vestibular-nuclear complex. The vestibulo-ocular reflex (VOR) provides visual focus on an object during head movements. The VOR arc between the vestibular system and the extraocular muscles performs this function. All semicircular canals and otolith organs have VOR arcs. The VOR keeps the visual image stable on the retina when the head moves. While the head is turned to the right, the VOR slowly turns the eyes to the left, and the reticular formation that tries to pull the eye to the midline also pulls the eye to the middle, this is called physiological nystagmus. Nystagmus may occur due to physiological (caloric, rotation chair, head shake) or pathology. The connections between the vestibular nuclei and the spinal cord create the vestibulo-spinal reflex (VSR). The VSR is responsible for maintaining posture. The lateral vestibulospinal tract originates from the lateral vestibular nucleus and extends to the spinal cord. It keeps the body upright by managing the head, trunk, and lower extremities against the slope using utricular input. The medial vestibulospinal tract originates from the medial, lateral, and inferior vestibular nuclei. It controls head movements with the inputs from the saccule. The vestibular nuclear complex is also connected with the contralateral vestibular nuclear complex, the brain stem centers controlling visceral reflexes, the cerebral cortex, and the hippocampus [2–4].

Vestibular system disorders can be central or peripheral. Peripheral vestibular system diseases as unilaterally or bilaterally, sudden or gradual, stable, progressive or fluctuating, temporarily or permanently, and completely or partially affect the vestibular receptor functions. Unilateral peripheral vestibular disorders disrupt the symmetry of input from vestibular sensors at the level of the brainstem. This may lead to disorientation in the perception of head movements and vestibular reflexes [2, 5].

Asymmetric vestibular inputs at the level of the vestibular nuclear complex may lead to static vestibular symptoms in the acute period and dynamic vestibular symptoms in the sub-acute and chronic period of the pathology. Static vestibular symptoms are nystagmus, vertigo, subjective visual vertical and horizontal perception disorientations, skew deviation, head and trunk tilt to the ipsilesional side, and neuro-vegetative symptoms. These symptoms occur spontaneously. In the ideal conditions, completely compensated in a few months. Dynamic vestibular symptoms are decreased and asymmetrical vestibulo-ocular reflex, vertigo, ocular counter rolling, postural instabilities, and cognitive symptoms. These symptoms occur during head movements. Compensation takes a longer time than static symptoms. It may not disappear completely [1, 6].

2. Vestibular compensation

It is a recovery mechanism after unilateral peripheral vestibulopathy. It is the central nervous system process that occurs to reduce the neural firing asymmetry at the level of the brainstem due to the lesion and to readjust the gain. In the process of regulation of peripheral function, mechanisms such as regulation of vestibular processing at the level of the brainstem, use of prediction and modulation of other senses instead of vestibular input, and adaptation to reduce the use of vestibular input are utilized. On the lesion side, the intrinsic excitability of the vestibular nuclei is increased, they are desensitized to inhibitory inputs, and their activity is gradually increased. The contralesional region is under the inhibitory effect of the cerebellum. Mechanisms involved in recovery after acute peripheral vestibular pathology with vestibular compensation, spontaneous recovery of damaged receptors and neurons, adaptation of residual vestibular function (the ability to adapt to head movement during the movement of an image on the retina), substitution for lost vestibular functions (with visual and somatosensory cues) and habituation to unwanted sensations (reduction of symptoms and pathological responses to provocative stimuli by systematic exposure to that stimulus). All of these mechanisms start simultaneously after the lesion. Achievement levels can affect each other. The success of one mechanism may obviate the need for the other. This results in the recovery processes being different from person to person. Static symptoms may improve within weeks, some of the dynamic symptoms may persist for life depending on the character of the disease. Otolytic symptoms resolve in a shorter time than semicircular canal symptoms. Vestibular compensation of static symptoms begins in the first 24–72 hours after acute unilateral peripheral vestibular lesion. The patient can walk with or without assistance after approximately 48 hours and starts to return to normal activities in two weeks. After the first three months, many patients can recover with minor static or dynamic symptoms. Static and dynamic symptoms continue to exist in vestibular compensation deficiencies. Factors affecting vestibular compensation directly or indirectly are age, type of vestibular pathology (stable/progressive/fluctuant), central nervous system function, lack of sensory input (vision, sense of touch), vestibulosuppressant use, musculoskeletal diseases (lower extremities or spine), sedentary lifestyle, poor head-eye stabilization, disturbances in the perception of stability, poor balance strategies, psychological disorders [7].

2.1 Why is vestibular compensation important?

The prevalence of vestibular diseases is high (35.4% over 40 years old, 64.8% over 60 years old, 84.8% over 80 years old), they increase the risk of falling, increase the cost of health care, decrease the quality of life, increase job loss, cause anxiety and depression. Recovery is not the same for every patient. Vestibular compensation can occur in three ways: full compensation, partial compensation, and decompensation. Symptoms of varying degrees of inadequate vestibular compensation are imbalance, impairment of visual fixation, spatial disorientation, vertigo, oscillopsia, sensitivity to environmental movements, cognitive problems, anxiety, and poor concentration. The consequences of these symptoms are inactivity, fear of falling, financial dependency, social isolation, disabilities in daily living activities/dependency, and decreased quality of life [1, 8].

3. Vestibular rehabilitation

It is a patient-oriented and exercise-based therapy program designed to support vestibular compensation after vestibular pathology. It benefits from vestibular adaptation, oculomotor movements, visual cues, somatosensory cues, postural strategies, and habituation while supporting vestibular healing mechanisms. Visual fixation exercises, head and eye movements combined with various activities, different upper extremity, head and trunk movements while maintaining balance despite reduced support surface, systematic repetition of movements that increase vertigo, and gradually exposing patients to various sensory or motor stimuli are used in the exercise program. The purposes of vestibular rehabilitation are to increase gaze stability, increase postural stability, reduce vertigo and the risk of falling, make the patient independent by improving the activities of daily living, and psychosocial well-being, and increase the health-related quality of life. In short, it is aimed to bring the patient closer to the normal state before the disease at the maximum level by increasing the safe movement and reducing the symptoms. It is an exercise-based therapy program designed to support vestibular compensation after vestibular pathology [8–12].

3.1 Indications of vestibular rehabilitation and patient selection

Vestibular rehabilitation is indicated for stable but decompensated vestibular lesions, regardless of the age of the patient, cause of pathology, duration, and intensity of symptoms. Stable and insufficiently compensated unilateral vestibular lesions, bilateral vestibular lesions, central vestibular lesions, mixed (central and peripheral) vestibular lesions, head trauma, psychogenic vertigo, age-related dizziness (with the aim of reducing the risk of falling), vertigo of unknown etiology, benign paroxysmal positional vertigo (for residual imbalance present in 2/3 of patients after a successful repositioning maneuver) benefit from vestibular rehabilitation. Vestibular compensation cannot develop in patients with active labyrinth pathology and fluctuating/progressive pathologies (Meniere's disease, perilymph fistula, superior semicircular canal dehiscence, enlarged vestibular aqueduct). Vestibulospressant use, visual and somatosensory deprivation, long-term immobilization, advanced age, and central nervous system lesions may prolong the recovery period, but do not completely prevent compensation [12, 13].

3.2 Vestibular rehabilitation methods

Conventional vestibular rehabilitation methods include Cawthorne-Cooksey exercises, multimodal Cawthorne-Cooksey exercises, vestibulo-ocular reflex adaptation exercises, habituation exercises, substitution exercises, and static and dynamic balance exercises [14, 15]. Alternative vestibular rehabilitation methods include augmented sensory feedback, movable platforms, full-screen optokinetic exercises, computer games (exergames), and virtual-reality-based vestibular rehabilitation. Alternative vestibular rehabilitation methods can be applied instead of conventional exercises or in combination with them. It can be preferred in patients who do not benefit from conventional methods.

The conventional vestibular rehabilitation program should be specific to the patient's complaints, suitable for lifestyle, consisting of a reasonable number and variety of exercises, easily learned, developed from easy to difficult-from simple to complex, functional, and individual. The steps of the rehabilitation program consist of evaluation, training of the patient and family, planning of the exercise program, domestic arrangements to increase the safety of movement, suggestions for the selection of assistive walking equipment and shoes if necessary, implementation of the exercise program, evaluation after the therapy, termination of the therapy and clinical follow-up.

The evaluation should consist of vestibular function tests (video head impulse, functional head impulse, subjective visual verticality and horizontality, static or dynamic posturography) that can evaluate vestibular involvement and compensation with numerical data and special scales that subjectively evaluate the patient's quality of life or limitations. The vestibular rehabilitation evaluation protocol, which consists of qualitative and quantitative data, helps to establish the exercise program, to support the belief and motivation of the patient in the rehabilitation program, to measure the success of treatment, to compare or prove the effectiveness of different rehabilitation methods, and to make the decision to terminate the rehabilitation program of the patient [11, 12].

Conventional exercises can be started with visual fixation exercises combined with head movements to support the vestibulo-ocular reflex. It can be done lying down, sitting, standing, or combined with walking, depending on the functional status of the patient. Saccadic and smooth pursuit movements are also added to the program in bilateral or central vestibular pathologies where substitution is required. The vestibulo-spinal reflex should also be supported to improve postural stability. In accordance with the functional status of the patient, a static posture should be practiced with a regular stance, two feet together, tandem or single leg on stable ground, movable ground, or foam. This should be followed by walking exercises, stepping forward, backward, left and right, and turning around by stepping around. Normal gait, straight gait, gait with horizontal and vertical movements of the head, and gait on the foam should be practiced. Turning activities should also be added to dynamic exercises. Static and dynamic balance exercises can also be applied by making changes in the visual input [11–13, 15].

Habituation exercises should be applied to the patient to reduce vertigo caused by movement. A program consisting of movements that the patient is most uncomfortable with can be created. While sitting or standing, repetitive head movements, trunk rotation, forward bending, and reaching up can be performed. A program consisting of exercises that will not cause neurovegetative symptoms should be established [11, 12, 15].

In conventional vestibular rehabilitation, the difficulty level of the exercises should be moderate or moderate-high. The exercises that the patient does very easily are non-functional exercises for vestibular compensation. The movements that are difficult at the beginning should be gradually made more difficult as they are performed more comfortably. Exercises can be applied in the clinic or as a home program when the patient comes for control at least once a week. In both methods, the patient should do at least two sets of vestibular exercises a day, and each set should last about half an hour. In addition to vestibular complaints that occur with movement, patients with neurovegetative complaints should do habituation exercises before meals. Exercises should be done in front of a wall or in corners to prevent falls. In addition to the exercise program, daily walking, simple sports activities, cognitive exercises, and regular reading activities should be added to the program. It would be appropriate for the patient not to use vestibulo-suppressants during the vestibular rehabilitation process.

Virtual reality (VR) is an important contribution of computer technology to the vestibular field in recent years. VR is a computer-generated simulation of a visual environment or an activity [16] and is defined as the user entering an interactive environment that mimics reality [17]. At the same time, VR can be defined as using computer technology to create simulations of objects, space, and events. It can represent both a real and a fictional world. This created virtual world includes not only visual content but also auditory and tactile stimuli and allows interaction with the user [8]. VR often uses a task to engage the user/patient in the system. This task can be walking through a crowded subway station, keeping an airplane on the desired route, completing the shopping list at the grocery store, painting an object, skiing, or tracking/capturing a target. In the VR system, the floor can be movable or fixed. In both cases, it is very important to prevent the patient from falling during exercise. Among the factors affecting the success of conventional vestibular rehabilitation are the patients' doing the exercises incorrectly, the active participation of the patients, and the need for their motivation. VR is an enjoyable and motivating method against the time-consuming, repetitive and monotonous conventional vestibular rehabilitation that makes it difficult for the patient to participate. VR-based vestibular rehabilitation is an enjoyable method for patients as it includes games that include real-time simulations, interactive functions, adaptation, substitution, and habituation exercises [2, 11, 14, 18].

Before VR, the use of technological equipment for vestibular rehabilitation started with exergames, which were reflected on TV screens and provided patient participation. With developments in the gaming industry, technologies have been added that combine an accelerometer and a force plate to provide visual and auditory feedback of patients' baseline pressure centers [19]. At the same time, computer games connected to the motion sensor were added [14]. In addition to these, optokinetic stimulation or creating a virtual environment by attaching smartphones to the head for use in the home environment has also been utilized [20–22].

Systems called real VR are immersive systems. Virtual reality immersion is the perception of one's physical existence in a non-physical world. This perception is created by surrounding the VR system user with visual, sound, or tactile stimuli that provide an immersive environment. In rehabilitation, the user's movements are detected and monitored by the system. It is a widely practiced technique for creating a virtual environment using a variety of spherical, flat screen, or head-mounted display formats. The user can interact with objects in VR using body movement. VR has recently gained popularity in medicine with the rapid development of mobile and visual technologies. It is used as an adjunct in psychiatry, in the treatment of anxiety, schizophrenia, or post-traumatic stress disorder, and in the treatment of cognitive disorders, Alzheimer's disease, Parkinson's disease, post-stroke hemiplegia, analgesic treatment of burns, pediatrics, cerebral palsy rehabilitation, and treatment of children with autism spectrum disorders [8, 14, 23, 24].

VR can provide visual, auditory, and tactile feedback that can motivate patients in vestibular rehabilitation, create a sense of physical presence in the virtual world, and provide personalized training. The system provides a hierarchical and customized presentation of realistic environmental stimuli adapted to patients' balance development [22]. Additional hardware can be added to monitor motion kinematics or provide force simulations and haptic feedback to participants [15]. The tactile feedback makes a significant contribution to vestibular rehabilitation, especially in upper extremity activities combined with trunk exercises and moving platform activities (for example, archery or skiing). Tactile feedback not only makes the activity more realistic and enjoyable but also strengthens proprioceptive input.

Fixed or mobile force plates or treadmills can be integrated into head-mounted VR systems. Head-mounted VE systems are very effective in improving vestibulo-ocular reflex, oculomotor movements, eye tracking, and head-eye coordination. Systems that cannot be integrated with any platform, requiring only eye or head movements or staying still, can be called "passive VR rehabilitation systems," systems that require providing or maintaining postural balance on a moving floor, stepping on a stable floor, walking on a treadmill or doing yoga can be called "active VR rehabilitation systems" [11, 15, 17, 19].

No photographs were used in this chapter for preventing to highlighting any VR system brand. The categories of VR-based vestibular rehabilitation exercises can be defined as:

1. Environment or condition simulations: Boat, automobile, airplane, escalator, metro station, and elevator simulations in devices with stable floors are very effective for habituation in patients who cannot tolerate crowded or active environments. Patients exposed to the active environment may show neurovegetative symptoms in the early period. Fear, panic, and a feeling of being away from the environment may occur. The number, speed, and visual characteristics of the parameters in the simulation should be started at a level that can be tolerated by the patient and gradually become more complicated. Simulation should be applied first in sitting, then in standing position on hard or soft ground in the following period. In unilateral peripheral vestibulopathy, especially if the vestibulo-ocular reflex gain is very low, patients are clearly uncomfortable with the motion simulations when they turn their heads towards the pathological side, motion simulation by changing the head position is very useful in these patients. In systems where the ground is mobile, simulations of subway stations, boats or waves are more difficult exercises as they also require the preservation of postural balance during visual mobility.

2. Optokinetic simulations: Images created using horizontal, vertical, or rotatory moving points, planets, or other different shapes. Background, size, number, movement speed, and direction of objects can be adjusted according to the patient's tolerance. In fixed systems, it can be worked in sitting and standing. In systems with a movable platform, ground motion also allows the patient to try to control posture while watching moving objects.

3. Head-eye coordination: They are used as adaptation and substitution exercises as they support both oculomotor movements, head movements, and vestibulo-ocular reflex. Managing the movements of an object (for example, an airplane, planet, or bird) with head movements, watching the moving object with head movements, focusing on the target where it turns the head, trying to find the materials given as a task in the market environment from the shelves can be given as examples of exercises in this category. Movement speed, locations, and sizes of objects can be changed according to the patient. Vestibular pathology causes patients to restrict their head movements. These exercises activate the patients' head and eye movements. These exercises can be done in systems with a fixed floor, again depending on the level of the patient, while sitting or standing on a hard floor or foam. They can also be combined with moving platforms.

4. Exercises involving upper extremity: Exercises involving upper extremity movements in vestibular rehabilitation are very important as they require trunk movements or stepping on motionless platforms. The sensors held by the patients in both hands can be used for shooting arrows, popping balloons, or painting objects. These exercises involve bending forward, reaching up, turning back, or stepping. Parameters of the simulation can be changed in accordance with the patient. Items that increase cognitive activity can be added to exercises.

5. Activity simulations: These exercises are used very effectively, especially in systems with moving platforms. For example, ski simulation creates an effective dynamic balance exercise by adjusting almost all parameters of the visual environment, the task, and the movement according to the patient.

In the use of VR systems for vestibular rehabilitation, appropriate planning is required for the person and the functional level of the person. Vestibular assessment protocols are also known to be included in these systems, but will not be discussed in this section.

In studies in the literature, VR has been used together with or as an alternative to the conventional method in vestibular pathologies. There are also studies comparing the two methods with each other. Compared to conventional vestibular rehabilitation, there are studies stating that the functional effects are the same, as well as studies stating that the satisfaction level of patients is higher in the VR group [6, 8, 14–16, 18, 19, 21–25].

The systems and protocols applied to differ between studies. The use of computer games, which do not fully comply with virtual reality, and even the use of force plate home systems have also been evaluated in this category by some researchers, but as studies have increased, research with real VR systems has diverged. The reasons for using smartphones or force plate systems are to reduce costs and to enable patients to exercise at home by using computer systems. VR systems are applied in the clinic. VR-based vestibular rehabilitation protocols have been applied in various ways in publications. VR sessions were applied in the clinic for 30–40 minutes five days a week or 35–45 minutes two days a week. In some protocols, home exercises are included in the program [17].

The VR system needs standardization of exercise protocols and assessment tools. Especially in head-mounted systems, cybersickness caused by the inability of patients to tolerate the image should be evaluated, the side effects of virtual environment use should be documented, and algorithms are needed to decide which patients are suitable for the conventional program and which patients are suitable for the VR program. Only validated methods should be used to evaluate rehabilitation success, both functionally and with questionnaires. In the rehabilitation program, the number and duration of sessions and the duration of sessions should be documented. Special assessment tools should be used to evaluate side effects such as cybersickness caused by virtual reality. Complications of virtual reality rehabilitation, such as falls and fractures, should be documented. Patients' use of symptom-suppressing drugs should be documented during the period of VR. Since VR cost systems are high, it is recommended to determine session costs [15, 16, 26].

VR-based vestibular rehabilitation combined with conventional vestibular exercises is a very effective method. Home exercises must be included in the protocol. It is known that patients who do home exercises regularly recover in a shorter time. It may be preferable to include virtual reality in the program after conventional exercises, safe standing, and walking are gained in the first few weeks for patients to gain the habit of doing regular vestibular exercises at home and for movement safety [2]. In protocols implemented using only VR or similar systems from the beginning of the rehabilitation program, the patient may misunderstand that he or she should exercise with only one device. The main thing in vestibular rehabilitation is the active participation of the patient and increasing his activity in the living area. Basically, vestibular rehabilitation is not a device-based method, it is a movement-based method. VR is an important part of the conventional vestibular rehabilitation protocol.

Advantages of conventional vestibular rehabilitation program are as follows:

- Vestibular rehabilitation is basically an equipment-free therapy method. Equipment is only an auxiliary tool.
- Conventional vestibular rehabilitation is a cost-effective and practical method.
- It strengthens the communication and cooperation between the patient and the clinician.
- It gives the patient the habit of exercising regularly in the living area.
- It ensures the active participation of the patients in the rehabilitation process.

Advantages of the virtual reality-based vestibular rehabilitation program are as follows:

- Enjoyable
- Motivating
- It can create a real-life perception as it completely covers the visual field

- Provides an effective habituation in patients who cannot tolerate environmental movement
- It can simulate special environments that cannot be achieved in clinical conditions
- The floor can be movable or fixed
- The amount of movement on the moving floor can be adjusted
- Provides the opportunity to gradually complicate the exercise

4. Conclusions

If the imbalance continues after vestibular disease, the patient should definitely be included in the vestibular rehabilitation program. Conventional vestibular rehabilitation methods enable the patient and family to be informed about both pathology and vestibular rehabilitation.

The patient should actively participate in the vestibular rehabilitation process. Home exercises are the most important part of vestibular rehabilitation. The patient should do at least one session of vestibular exercises every day. They should continue these exercises on the days they do not come to the clinic.

Vestibular rehabilitation is a patient-centered approach, not an instrument-oriented approach. Of course, virtual-reality systems are unrivaled in terms of the use of conditions that cannot be provided in the clinic within the scope of the rehabilitation program. Conventional vestibular rehabilitation methods are not sufficient to gain tolerance to external motion, especially in motion sickness patients.

In the clinic, starting the vestibular rehabilitation program with conventional exercises and continuing the program with virtual reality after the patient gains the ability to move safely is very effective in terms of strengthening the patient's active participation in the program and patient-clinician communication.

Vestibular rehabilitation is an exercise-based therapy program designed to support central compensation after vestibular pathology. While supporting vestibular compensation mechanisms: it benefits from vestibular adaptation, oculomotor movements, visual cues, somatosensory cues, postural strategies, and habituation. The aims of vestibular rehabilitation are to increase gaze and postural stability, to reduce vertigo and fall risk, and to make the patient independent by improving daily living activities and psychosocial well-being.

Recently, computer games augmented reality and virtual reality systems have been used in vestibular rehabilitation programs with the developing computer technology. In particular, augmented and virtual reality systems enable the patient to perform challenging visual conditions and special activities in a controlled manner which cannot be provided in standard clinical conditions. In this chapter, a literature review is presented about the roles of classical vestibular rehabilitation and virtual reality systems in improving vestibular compensation.

Acknowledgements

I would like to thank Prof. Dr. M. Tayyar Kalcioglu for his collaboration and contributions.

The author declares that no funding has been provided during the preparation of this book chapter.

Conflict of interest

The author declares no conflict of interest.

Author details

Başak Mutlu
Faculty of Health Sciences, Department of Audiology, Istanbul Medeniyet University, Istanbul, Turkey

*Address all correspondence to: basakogun@yahoo.com

References

[1] Lacour M, Bernard-Demanze L. Interaction between vestibular compensation mechanisms and vestibular rehabilitation therapy: 10 recommendations for optimal functional recovery. Frontiers in Neurology. 2015;**5**:285

[2] Xie M, Zhou K, Patro N, Chan T, Levin M, Gupta MK, et al. Virtual reality for vestibular rehabilitation: A systematic review. Otology & Neurotology. 2021;**42**(7):967-977

[3] Kingma H, van de Berg R. Anatomy, physiology, and physics of the peripheral vestibular system. Handbook of Clinical Neurology. 2016;**137**:1-16

[4] Ferrè ER, Haggard P. Vestibular cognition: State-of-the-art and future directions. Cognitive Neuropsychology. 2020;**37**(7-8):413-420

[5] Curthoys IS, Halmagyi M. Vestibular compensation: Clinical changes in vestibular function with time after unilateral vestibular loss. In: Herdman SJ, editor. Vestibular Rehabilitation. 3rd ed. Philadelphia: F.A. Davis Co.; 2007. pp. 172-194

[6] Alahmari KA, Sparto PJ, Marchetti GF, Redfern MS, Furman JM, Whitney SL. Comparison of virtual reality-based therapy with customized vestibular physical therapy for the treatment of vestibular disorders. IEEE Transactions on Neural Systems and Rehabilitation Engineering. 2014;**22**(2):389-399

[7] Lacour M, Helmchen C, Vidal PP. Vestibular compensation: The neuro-otologist's best friend. Journal of Neurology. 2016;**263**(Suppl. 1):S54-S64

[8] Stankiewicz T, Gujski M, Niedzielski A, Chmielik LP. Virtual reality vestibular rehabilitation in 20 patients with vertigo due to peripheral vestibular dysfunction. Medical Science Monitor. 2020;**26**:e930182

[9] Herdman SJ. Vestibular rehabilitation. Current Opinion in Neurology. 2013;**26**(1):96-101

[10] Arnold SA, Stewart AM, Moor HM, Karl RC, Reneker JC. The effectiveness of vestibular rehabilitation interventions in treating unilateral peripheral vestibular disorders: A systematic review. Physiotherapy Research International. 2017;**22**:3

[11] Hall CD, Herdman SJ, Whitney SL, Anson ER, Carender WJ, Hoppes CW, et al. Vestibular rehabilitation for peripheral vestibular hypofunction: An updated clinical practice guideline from the Academy of Neurologic Physical Therapy of the American Physical Therapy Association. Journal of Neurologic Physical Therapy. 2022;**46**(2):118-177

[12] Sulway S, Whitney SL. Advances in vestibular rehabilitation. Advances in Oto-Rhino-Laryngology. 2019;**82**:164-169

[13] Han BI, Song HS, Kim JS. Vestibular rehabilitation therapy: Review of indications, mechanisms, and key exercises. Journal of Clinical Neurology. 2011;**7**(4):184-196

[14] Rosiak O, Krajewski K, Woszczak M, Jozefowicz-Korczynska M. Evaluation of the effectiveness of a Virtual Reality-based exercise program for unilateral peripheral vestibular deficit. Journal of Vestibular Research. 2018;**28**(5-6):409-415

[15] Bergeron M, Lortie CL, Guitton MJ. Use of virtual reality tools for vestibular disorders rehabilitation: A comprehensive analysis. Advance Medicine. 2015;**2015**:916735

[16] Tychsen L, Foeller P. Effects of immersive virtual reality headset viewing on young children: Visuomotor function, postural stability, and motion sickness. American Journal of Ophthalmology. 2020;**209**:151-159

[17] Heffernan A, Abdelmalek M, Nunez DA. Virtual and augmented reality in the vestibular rehabilitation of peripheral vestibular disorders: Systematic review and meta-analysis. Scientific Reports. 2021;**11**(1):17843

[18] Micarelli A, Viziano A, Augimeri I, Micarelli D, Alessandrini M. Three-dimensional head-mounted gaming task procedure maximizes effects of vestibular rehabilitation in unilateral vestibular hypofunction: A randomized controlled pilot trial. International Journal of Rehabilitation Research. 2017;**40**(4):325-332

[19] Meldrum D, Herdman S, Moloney R, Murray D, Duffy D, Malone K, et al. Effectiveness of conventional versus virtual reality based vestibular rehabilitation in the treatment of dizziness, gait and balance impairment in adults with unilateral peripheral vestibular loss: A randomised controlled trial. BMC Ear, Nose, and Throat Disorders. 2012;**12**:3

[20] Soltani P, Andrade R. The influence of virtual reality head-mounted displays on balance outcomes and training paradigms: A systematic review. Front Sports Act Living. 2021;**2**:531535

[21] Mandour AE, El-Gharib AM, Emara AA, Elmahallawy TH. Virtual reality versus optokinetic stimulation in visual vertigo rehabilitation. European Archives of Oto-Rhino-Laryngology. 2022;**279**(3):1609-1614

[22] Hsu SY, Fang TY, Yeh SC, Su MC, Wang PC, Wang VY. Three-dimensional, virtual reality vestibular rehabilitation for chronic imbalance problem caused by Ménière's disease: A pilot study. Disability and Rehabilitation. 2017;**39**(16):1601-1606

[23] Yeh SC, Huang MC, Wang PC, Fang TY, Su MC, Tsai PY, et al. Machine learning-based assessment tool for imbalance and vestibular dysfunction with virtual reality rehabilitation system. Computer Methods and Programs in Biomedicine. 2014;**116**(3):311-318

[24] Yeh SC, Chen S, Wang PC, Su MC, Chang CH, Tsai PY. Interactive 3-dimensional virtual reality rehabilitation for patients with chronic imbalance and vestibular dysfunction. Technology and Health Care. 2014;**22**(6):915-921

[25] Kanyılmaz T, Topuz O, Ardıç FN, Alkan H, Öztekin SNS, Topuz B, et al. Effectiveness of conventional versus virtual reality-based vestibular rehabilitation exercises in elderly patients with dizziness: A randomized controlled study with 6-month follow-up. Brazilian Journal of Otorhinolaryngology. 2021;**2021**:S1808

[26] Groth C, Tauscher JP, Heesen N, Hattenbach M, Castillo S, Magnor M. Omnidirectional galvanic vestibular stimulation in virtual reality. IEEE Transactions on Visualization and Computer Graphics. 2022;**28**(5): 2234-2244

Chapter 6

Hearing and Vestibular Testing in Menière's Disease

Moslem Shaabani

Abstract

Endolymphatic hydrops (ELH) known as the main pathophysiology of Menière's disease (MD) changes both the cochlear and vestibular function of the inner ear. These physiological changes can occur simultaneously (cochleovestibular involvement) or separately (cochlear or vestibular involvement). They can also present unilaterally or bilaterally (simultaneously or sequentially). Moreover, ELH recurs periodically without any specific etiology and known rhythm. Therefore, the patient referred for audiological tests may be in attack phase (acute) or inter-attack phase (chronic). MD itself may be in early- or advanced stage. In addition, considering comorbidity (vestibular or non-vestibular) is vital for differential diagnosis. On the other hand, each audiological test (including PTA, ECochG, VNG, vHIT, SVV, VEMPs ...) has its specific diagnostic viewpoint and gives us a limited snapshot of MD's clinical picture. Consequently, in this chapter, we want to discuss these viewpoints and try to explain associations and dissociations of audiological test findings in MD patients.

Keywords: endolymphatic hydrops, pure-tone audiometry, videonystagmography, electrocochleography, video head impulse test, subjective visual vertical, vestibular evoked myogenic potential

1. Introduction

Menière's disease (MD) is an inner ear (or labyrinthine) disease [1]. It described by a French physician, Prosper Ménière, in 1861. Through observing a group of patients, he realized that symptoms such as spells of spontaneous vertigo attacks, occurrence of positional vertigo between attacks, tinnitus, and hearing fluctuations that do not necessarily occur together might be the clinical picture of a single disease. He was the first to emphasize that vertigo could be caused by a damage to the inner ear [2].

As an ear disease, with episodic vertigo and fluctuating aural symptoms (hearing, tinnitus, or fullness) [3], MD patients usually referred to audiology (or vertigo) clinics. However, we know that each audiological test has its specific diagnostic viewpoint. Therefore, each test shows us a snapshot of real disease.

MD can present in one or both ears (simultaneously or sequentially). Moreover, it is not a stable disease; it usually occurs in "attack-inter attack pattern" (i.e., it relapses) and progresses to different parts of inner ear (s) (i.e., cochlea, semicircular canals, saccule, or utricle). In each attack, new destruction or distortion can occur [4]. Hence, the perspective of inner ear changes after each attack. This scene may return to previous state in inter-attack period.

Does destruction occur the same for all parts of inner ear(s)? Does recovery happen the same for all parts of inner ear(s)? What is the best time for testing the patient after the attack? What are the best tests to achieve the diagnosis? Do we have specific and sensitive tests for diagnosing the hydrops in each part of inner ear?

In the following, we discuss the viewpoint achieved by each audiological test and try to explain associations and dissociations of their findings in MD patients.

2. General auditory viewpoint

2.1 Introduction on pathophysiology and auditory tests

Endolymphatic hydrops (ELH) is the main pathophysiology of MD affects hydrodynamics of inner ear fluids [5]. As a result, it changes the mass and stiffness (as well as the resonance frequency) of labyrinthine compartment. We expect that cochlear hydrops resulted in auditory and aural symptoms such as hearing loss, tinnitus, fullness, and hyperacusis (vestibular hydrops discussed in the Section 3).

It seems that cochlear hydrops decreases the distance between stapes and endolymphatic space. The latter contains basilar membrane (BM), which holds outer hair cells (OHCs) and inner hair cells (IHCs). Thus, cochlear hydrops alter the activation of OHCs, IHCs and their afferents (and probably their efferents too). These alterations can explain auditory and aural symptoms of MD. Can we track the alterations (i.e., due to cochlear hydrops) using audiometry, otoacoustic emissions (OAEs), electrocochleography (ECochG), auditory brainstem response (ABR), or cochlear hydrops analysis masking procedure (CHAMP)?

On the other hand, cochlear hydrops increases the outward pressure on stapes and ossicular chain of middle ear. Accordingly, it changes the inner ear perspective concomitantly with changing the perspective of middle ear. Can we track these changed perspectives using a technique such as wide-band tympanometry (WBT)?

In the following sections, we want to sketch these auditory viewpoints about MD.

2.2 Audiometry and aural symptoms

We can consider general auditory profile (i.e., audiogram) as the main audiological test that aids in diagnosis and monitoring of MD. The Barany society (2015) introduces two categories for MD: definite and probable. Two or more episodes of spontaneous vertigo (lasting 20 min to 12–24 h) and fluctuating aural symptoms (hearing, tinnitus, or fullness) are common between two categories. Nevertheless, in definite MD patients, sensorineural hearing loss (SNHL) in low to mid audiometric frequencies, at least in one ear and on one occasion, is an additional diagnostic criterion [3]. Consequently, it seems vital to acquire periodic audiograms to diagnose the MD and its progression behavior.

Is there a specific pattern for hearing loss in this disease? What is the pattern of progress? Do we have a classification for different stages of the disease?

Several audiometric configurations are proposed in MD: peak audiogram (normal hearing in 2000 or 3000 Hz), rising (low frequency SNHL), falling (descending, or high frequency SNHL), trough, atypical notch (in 1 or 2 KHz, based on our experience; see **Figure 1**), and flat SNHL. In early stage of MD, peak and low-frequency audiograms are more common. However, in the advanced stage, flat audiogram (with or without more high-frequency loss) arises [6]. In AAO-HNS guidelines (1995), four stages of MD classified based on pure-tone audiometry average (PTA): stage I, <26 dB; stage II, 26–40 dB; stage III, 41–70 dB; stage IV, >70 dB [7].

In the course of disease, it seems that the hearing loss increases from about slight-to-mild (low-frequency SNHL) in early stage to moderate-to-severe (flat SNHL) in advanced stage. Some studies showed a significant correlation between the grade of hydrops and severity of hearing thresholds in low and mid audiometric frequencies. Moreover, the audiogram fluctuates with the average of 20–30 dB. The fluctuation

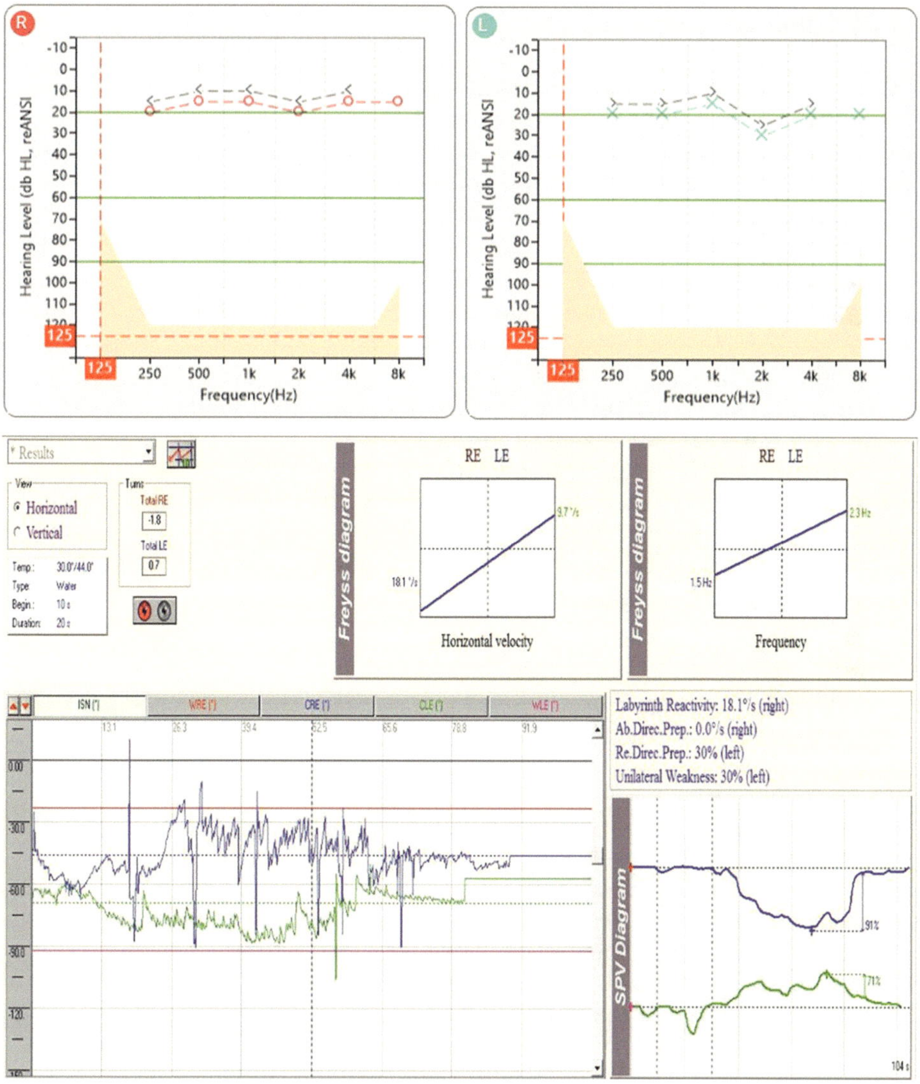

Figure 1.
Upper part: Audiogram of a female patient (52y) with 7 years' history of episodic vertigo attacks that occurred in every 2 months. As you can see, we have only a 2 KHz notch in the left ear (i.e., the ear with aural fullness and tinnitus). Lower part: The picture shows the caloric test results (SYNAPSYS VNG software by Inventis srl.). Caloric result of the same patient with significant vestibular weakness in the left ear (left-UW). Note. The patient had normal middle-ear function and normal vHIT results.

is more during the early stage (perhaps the first year following MD onset) and then subsides [1, 5, 6, 8]. The frequency of bilateral MD is about 2–47% [9].

2.3 Mechano-acoustic viewpoint

The ear is composed of three main parts: outer ear, middle ear, and inner ear. In these three parts, exactly before mechanoelectrical transduction by hair cells, we are facing with mechanical energy of incident sound power. Part of this power reflected back and part of that absorbed in the ear. We can track changes in power reflectance and power absorbance of the middle ear by wide-band tympanometry (WBT).

2.3.1 Wide-band tympanometry

WBT is a method for evaluating middle-ear diseases such as otitis media with effusion (OME), otosclerosis, and ossicular chain discontinuity. Compared to the traditional 226-Hz tympanometry, WBT uses multiple frequencies (ranging from to 8000 Hz) in 1/24 octave intervals through a descending pressure sweep (between +250 and − 350 daPa). Therefore, it is more sensitive to middle-ear transfer function [10, 11].

By increasing perilymphatic pressure, ELH can push the stapes footplate toward the middle ear. Thus, it restricts the movement of the ossicular chain and decreases the compliance of the middle ear [11]. This condition is almost similar to the OME (among other middle-ear pathologies). From another viewpoint, ELH decreases the impedance of cochlear part, just like large vestibular aqueduct syndrome (LVAS) (among other inner ear pathologies). Consequently, studies showed that resonance frequency of the middle ear decreased in MD [11], LVAS [12], and OME [13]. Moreover, power reflectance in high frequency range (2–4 KHz) increased in MD patients [14]. Therefore, WBT has opened a new window on inner-ear pathologies.

2.4 Electro-acoustic viewpoint

The cochlea emits some sounds spontaneously or in response to an external auditory stimulus. These sounds are called spontaneous otoacoustic emissions (SOAEs) or evoked OAEs (EOAEs), respectively.

2.4.1 Otoacoustic emissions

OAEs provide a tool for evaluating the function and integrity of outer hair cells (OHCs). Presence or absence of OAEs, their amplitudes in different frequencies, and suppression of them through contralateral noise are valuable cues for delineating OHC loss or dysfunction, estimation of audiogram, and testing auditory efferent system, respectively. Do these cues change in Ménière disease?

In MD patients, OAE features are usually compatible with the level of hearing loss. In other words, it does not differ from other patients with the same level of sensorineural hearing loss [15]. However, in some of MD patients with hearing level between 30 and 60 dB, OAEs are normally present. Based on these cases, it is possible that IHCs become involved sooner due to ELH [16]. On the other hand, a feature of OAE (or OHC function) that we have not yet evaluated or do not know may have changed in MD patients. A study by Murdin and cowerkers (2010) showed that DOPAE suppression is lower in patients with vestibular migraine [17].

Suppression of OAEs needs acetylcholine (Ach). Ach is inhibited by calcitonin gene-related peptide (CGRP) activity. Increased activity of CGRP in the migraineurs' inner ear could result in an abnormal OAE suppression [18]. Future studies will show whether we can use OAE suppression to differentiate between MD and vestibular migraine patients.

A case study by Chun and colleagues (2009) revealed that OAE recovery is a tool for monitoring treatment in patients with luetic endolymphatic hydrops (due to syphilis) [19]. Consequently, OAE features, OAE suppression, and OAE recovery provide important toolbox for evaluating and monitoring the diseases that involve inner ear.

2.5 Auditory electro-physiologic viewpoint

There are several electro-physiologic tests, which analyze auditory responses and contain good information for diagnosis of ELH. In this section, we discuss about electrocochleography (ECochG) and cochlear hydrops analysis masking procedure (CHAMP).

2.5.1 Electrocochleography (ECochG)

In ECochG test, we present an acoustic stimulus (usually click or tone burst) via a headphone (or insert phone) and record a two-component response through several leads (electrodes) around the ear (i.e., extratympanic method). One component originates from cochlear part, mainly inner hair cells (named summating potential or SP), and the other component evokes by auditory nerve fibers (named compound action potential or AP). The hypothesis is that ELH can deform basilar membrane and affect the latency and amplitude of these two components [20].

There are two ratio methods for analyzing ECochG results: 1. SP/AP amplitude ratio; and 2. SP/AP area ratio [21].

By defining latency and amplitude of SP and AP components, we can measure SP/AP amplitude ratio. For latency measurement, we need the stimulus onset (zero time); and for amplitude measurement, we need a baseline (BL). Enhancement of SP/AP amplitude ratio is a positive indicator for ELH [21] (**Figure 2**). Baba et al. (2009) reported 0.314 as upper limits of normal for SP/AP amplitude ratio [22]. Based on previous studies, it seems that the ratio of more than 0.37 (or less than 0.5 as stated by Gibson [23]) has a low sensitivity (less than 60%) but an acceptable specificity (around 90%) for diagnosing MD [20, 23]. Using 1-KHz tone burst and through transtympanic recording, which can make the response four times bigger, the audiologist can reach a higher sensitivity for diagnosing MD (around 79%) [23].

Several factors related to the subject (i.e., MD patient) affect the usefulness of this ratio that include being in attack or inter-attack phase, in early or advanced stage of disease, and the degree of hearing loss. Therefore, this criterion may only work in half of the MD patients [20].

Considering SP/AP area ratio can improve the sensitivity and specificity of the diagnosis. Baba et al. (2009) reported 1.56 as upper limits of normal for this ratio. They reported area ratio of 1.97 ± 0.55 in definite MD patients [22].

Finally, it should be noted that although the specificity of the ECochG results (the amplitude and area ratios) is high, but sometimes the test is positive in similar diseases such as superior semicircular dehiscence (SSCD) [24] and vestibular migraine [25].

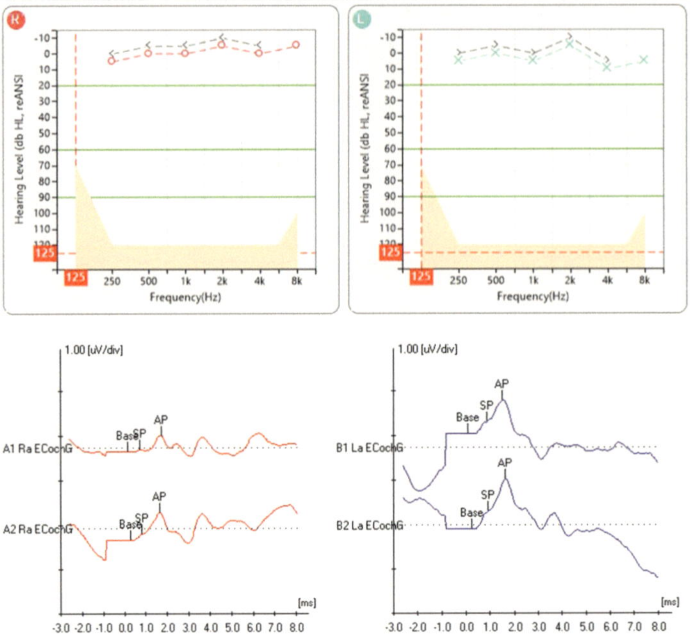

Figure 2.
Upper part: Audiogram of a female patient (39y) with 3 years' history of episodic vertigo attacks (in every 4–5 months) associated with nausea and left-ear tinnitus. She had normal audiogram and normal middle-ear function. Lower part: ECochG results. The amplitude ratio of SP/AP was 29% for A2-trace (normal ear) and 44% for B1-trace (disordered ear).

2.5.2 Cochlear hydrops analysis masking procedure (CHAMP)

ELH can affect the traveling wave velocity (TWV). Previous studies showed that TWV increases in MD patients [20]. By comparing wave V latency of auditory brainstem response (ABR) in response to click-only stimulus, and click-plus-high pass

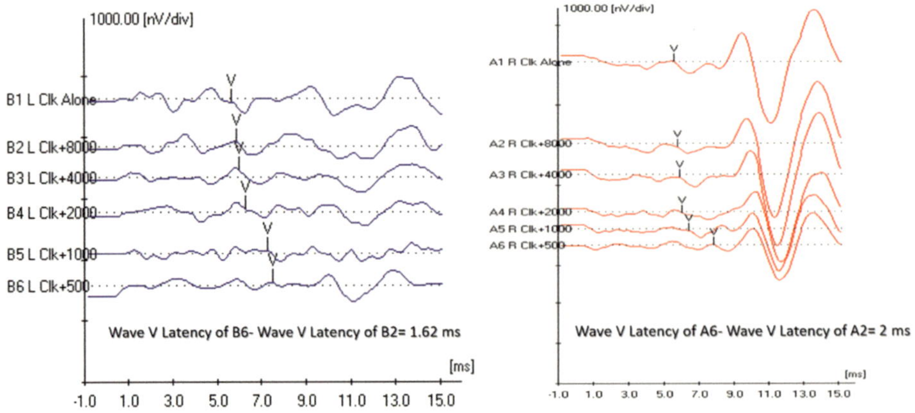

Figure 3.
CHAMP results of the patient presented in the **Figure 2***. Note the decreased difference between the wave V latency of basal part and that of apical part in the left ear with a history of MD.*

noises, we can measure the effect of increased TWV in MD patients. It means that different noises mask different parts of basilar membrane and permit us to differentiate the response of basal part of cochlea from its apical part.

Increased TWV resulted in decreased latency difference between the wave V latency of basal part and that of apical part (**Figure 3**). This is really occurs in MD patients. However, the CHAMP test has only high sensitivity and specificity in definite MD patients [26].

3. General vestibular viewpoint

ELH as the main pathophysiology of MD affects hydrodynamics of vestibular system (semicircular canals and two otolithic organs including utricle and saccule) too. We expect that vestibular hydrops resulted in vestibular symptoms such as dizziness, vertigo, nausea, vomiting, motion sensitivity, and imbalance.

It seems that vestibular hydrops changes the distance between cochlear and vestibular organs, as well as between inner ear and middle ear. Like as cochlear part, vestibular end organs have also specialized sensory cells including type I and type II hair cells. Thus, vestibular hydrops alters the activation of type I, type II and their afferents (and probably their efferents too). These alterations can explain vestibular symptoms of MD. We can categorize them as vestibulo-ocular and vestibulo-spinal symptoms mediated by neural pathways of vestibulo-ocular reflex (VOR) and vestibulo-spinal reflex (VSR), respectively. It is worthy to note that vestibulo-collic and vestibulo-sympathetic reflexes have important roles in balance system, too.

The vestibular system differs from auditory system in that the right and left vestibular systems have functional pairing. It means that they function as two interconnected scale pans. This intra-system connection (or functional pairing) exists in both peripheral vestibular system (from vestibules up to vestibular nuclei in brainstem) and central vestibular system (from vestibular nuclei toward cortical vestibular regions). Therefore, vestibular hydrops can affect this functional pairing. The pairing deficiency can track using cervical vestibular evoked myogenic potentials (cVEMP), ocular vestibular evoked myogenic potentials (oVEMP), videonystagmography (VNG), video head impulse test (vHIT), and subjective visual vertical/horizontal (SVV/AVH) tests.

Another unique feature of vestibular system is that it is a sensory input for our global balance system. Other sensory inputs for balance include visual and somatosensory ones. These three main inputs work as a whole-interconnected system to keep us balanced (i.e., we have inter-system functional pairing, too). Thus, vestibular hydrops can affect the global balance of the patient. Using posturography test, we can evaluate the balance of the MD patient.

In the following sections, we want to sketch these vestibular viewpoints about MD.

3.1 Vestibular electro-physiologic viewpoint

Interestingly, we can record the sound-evoked responses of the vestibular system by placing electrodes on the neck muscle (i.e., sternocleidomastoid muscle or SCM) or below the eyes (i.e., inferior oblique muscle). The former mode records cervical vestibular evoked myogenic potentials (cVEMP), and the latter mode records ocular vestibular evoked myogenic potentials (oVEMP).

3.1.1 Cervical vestibular evoked myogenic potentials (cVEMP)

cVEMP is a saccular response. Therefore, it evaluates the function of inferior vestibular nerve and sacculocollic reflex. cVEMP response is a biphasic electrophysiological response named p13-n23, based on the occurrence latency of each component [27, 28]. Recent study by Shahnaz and David (2021) on cVEMP that performed in supine position with raised and turned head showed normal latency range of 16 ± 1.08 ms for p1 and 24.6 ± 1.98 ms for n1 [29].

cVEMP is an ipsilateral inhibitory response. It means that presentation of each acoustic stimulus (usually click or 500 Hz tone burst) for example, to the right ear instantaneously decreases the tonus of contracted right SCM. This change induces a potential in the recording electrode placed on the SCM. The average of them in response to several stimuli (usually about 50–200 stimulus) creates p1-n1 response. Using BC stimulus (via a bone oscillator) can provoke a bilateral response. The exact placement of oscillator determines the latency and amplitude of each response [20, 30].

Usually, we record cVEMP unilaterally and compare the amplitude of responses (i.e., from the peak of p13 to trough of n23) recorded from each side (**Figure 4**). This analysis is called interaural asymmetry ratio (IAR). The upper limit of normal for IAR is about 0.4 [31]. In some reports, abnormal IAR is considered as more than 0.33 [32]. Based on IAR and the symptomatic ear (as well as historical background), we can define the augmented side (i.e., an increased VEMP response that indicated a hyperactive or hypersensitive saccule) or the reduced side (i.e., a decreased or absent VEMP response that indicated a hypoactive or hyposensitive saccule).

An increased and decreased/absent VEMP responses reported in the early and late stages of MD, respectively. Saccular hydrops and saccular degeneration proposed for explaining these results, respectively [27]. Moreover, interaural differences such as IAR and threshold difference between left and right VEMPs, usually affected by the fact that the asymptomatic (or unaffected) ear might have some abnormalities (i.e., subclinical MD). For pointing this problem, the tuning curve method suggested. In this method, amplitude of 500 Hz VEMP compared with that of 1000 Hz in the same ear [33]. The ratio decreased in MD patients (i.e., flattening of the tuning curve occurs because in hydropic

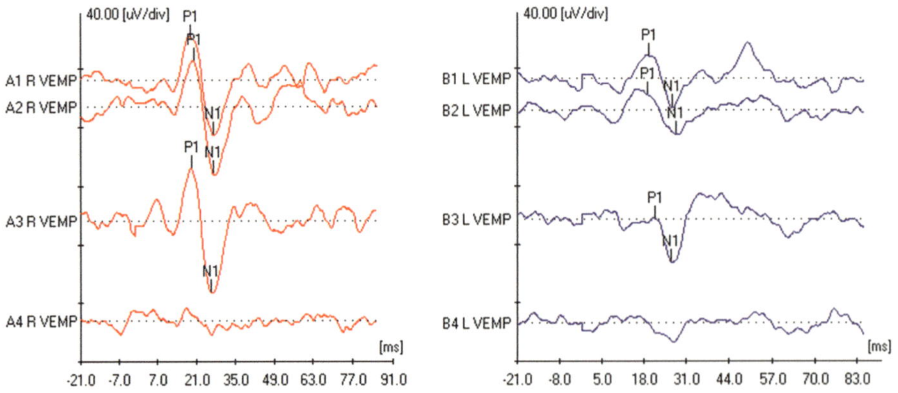

Figure 4.
cVEMP results of the patient presented in the **Figures 2** *and* **3**. *Note the interaural asymmetry ratio (IAR) of −48% (i.e., smaller VEMP response in the left ear with a history of MD).*

ear, endolymphatic tuning shifts to 100 Hz). They showed that this ratio could be a marker for MD progression because the ratio is high during acute phase and is normal during intermediate stable phase [33]. Of course, the ambiguity is whether we are going to use the test to determine the disorder or to use the test to grade the disorder we already know.

In any case, the point of specificity that mentioned above about ECochG raised again. cVEMP threshold is a suitable parameter for distinguishing SSCD from MD, but overlaps with vestibular migraine remains a clinical challenge [20].

3.1.2 Ocular vestibular evoked myogenic potentials (oVEMP)

oVEMP is an utricular response. Therefore, it evaluates the function of superior vestibular nerve and the utriculo-ocular reflex. oVEMP response is a biphasic electrophysiological response (n1-p1; n10-p15) [27, 34]. Recent study by Shahnaz and David (2021) with a new electrode montage named nasal alar montage found a shorter latency for n1 (12 ± 1.67 ms) and p1 (16 ± 1.72 ms) in comparison with traditional infraorbital montage [29].

oVEMP is a contralateral excitatory response provoked by excitation of contralateral inferior oblique muscle (re. stimulus ear). It should be noted that almost everything that was said about cVEMP in MD is true here for oVEMP as well [20, 30]. However, the different origins of these two VEMP responses can help us to differentiate vestibular disorders or to estimate the extent of the disease. In fact, it is better to record both responses, even with both AC and BC stimuli, to achieve the best clinical picture of the patient.

3.2 Vestibulo-ocular viewpoint

We know that the involuntary eye movements, which can occur due to head movements, follow vestibular stimulation (i.e., excitation and inhibition of both peripheral and central vestibular systems in the frames of intra-system and inter-system functional pairing). Therefore, unilateral vestibular disorder, or asymmetric bilateral vestibular disorder, can cause involuntary eye movements when the head is at rest. These eye movements are vestibular-evoked nystagmus.

Accordingly, by examining eye movements during head rest, head movements, or positioning the head, or while stimulating the vestibular system, for example, by thermal (caloric), vibrational, or electrical stimulation, the function of VOR reflex and the occurrence of abnormal eye movements (such as compensatory saccades or different types of nystagmi) can be examined. For this purpose, we use videonystagmography (VNG) test battery (SYNAPSYS VNG by Inventis srl) and video head impulse test (vHIT) (SYNAPSYS VHIT by Inventis srl).

The otolith system detects and provides us the real vertical axis of gravity. Based on this, and with the help of our real-world experiences from childhood, and the benefit of intra-system and inter-system pairings, we can understand other degrees of tilt in space; i.e., the tilt of ourselves, which can also be extended to the tilt of objects in our surrounding world. Our perception of the real vertical and horizontal axes is a manifestation of the balance in this complicated system. For testing this perception in general (and not precisely!), we can use subjective visual vertical/horizontal (SVV/SVH) tests.

3.2.1 Videonystagmography (VNG)

For performing VNG test battery, a goggle with infrared camera(s) placed over the patient's eyes. VNG test battery consists of two categories: 1. Central oculomotor tests that have a visual target and 2. Peripheral vestibular tests that do not have any target. The first category includes saccade, smooth pursuit, optokinetic, and gaze tests (here, we will not discuss their results for MD diagnosis). The second category includes spontaneous nystagmus test (SNT), head-shaking test (HST), Dix-Hallpike test (DHT), Positional test (PT), and Caloric test (CT). Instead of head shaking, we can use vestibular vibrator to assess vibration-induced nystagmus (VIN).

In peripheral tests, we are looking for abnormal nystagmus. Unilateral MD (or bilateral asymmetric MD), especially in the acute (or active) phase, can make an imbalance in vestibular system. This imbalance can manifest as spontaneous nystagmus (SN) (**Figure 5**). Bery et al. visited an interesting MD patient during vertigo attack and recorded initial "irritative" nystagmus that beats toward affected ear and after about 2 minutes of onset reverses its direction toward the unaffected ear ("paralytic" nystagmus) [35]. Following the latter nystagmus, and about 3 days after onset (or within the acute phase, a recovery nystagmus toward the affected ear can occur in some MD patients [35]. For that reason, in interpreting the results of SN, the audiologist should pay attention to the disease phase.

Moreover, the imbalance may exhibit itself as head-shaking nystagmus (HSN) (**Figure 6**). HSN is reported in about 68% of MD patients. However, HSN is more recordable in the acute phase and has a diverse direction. Its direction may be toward or away from the affected side or may be biphasic [36, 37]. Therefore, for its correct interpretation, the patient's symptoms and the results of other tests should be considered.

On the other hand, the imbalance may exhibit itself as VIN (**Figure 7**). VIN is reported in 28–71% of MD patients. It is often recordable in the acute phase and mostly as the irritative type (i.e., beating toward the affected ear) [38]. In our study on 29 patients with unilateral chronic MD tested in inter-attack phase, we found that vibrational stimulation of the affected ear with 100 Hz stimulus (mastoidal stimulation)

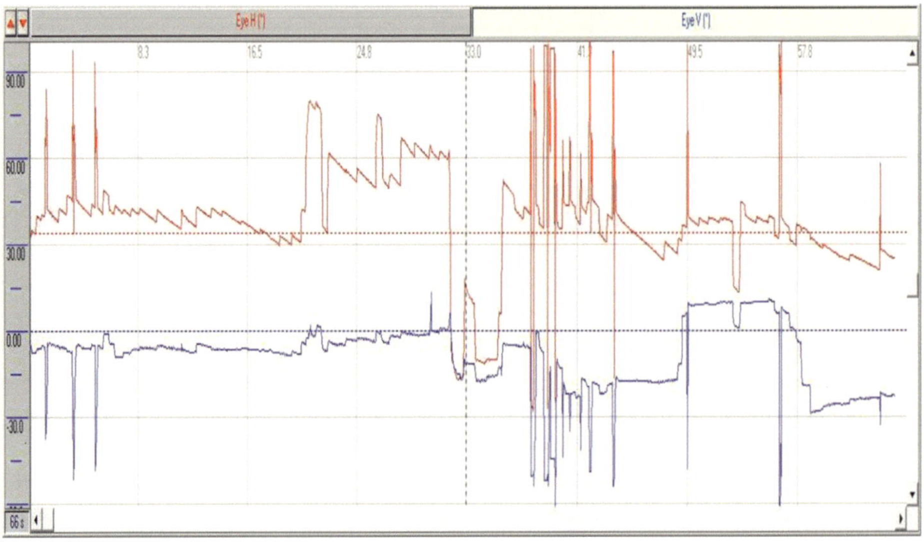

Figure 5.
The picture shows spontaneous nystagmus (SN) test results (SYNAPSYS VNG software by Inventis srl.) of a male patient (29y) with 5 years of MD symptoms in his right ear. Note the right-beating SN (with SPV of about 5 degree/seconds). His last attack occurred 2 days before recording this VNG test. This type of SN can be considered as recovery nystagmus. Please see the text for more discussion.

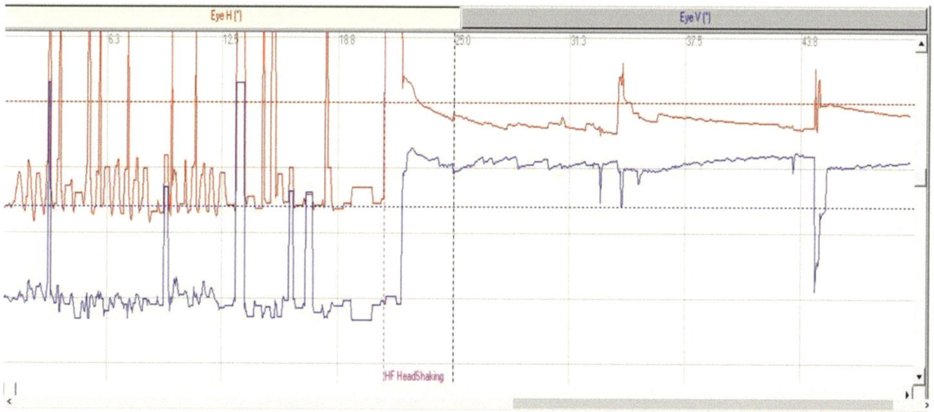

Figure 6.
The picture shows head-shaking nystagmus (HSN) test results (SYNAPSYS VNG software by Inventis srl.) of the patient presented in the **Figure 1**. *Note the right-down-beating HSN (with SPV of about 0.7 degree/seconds in both directions).*

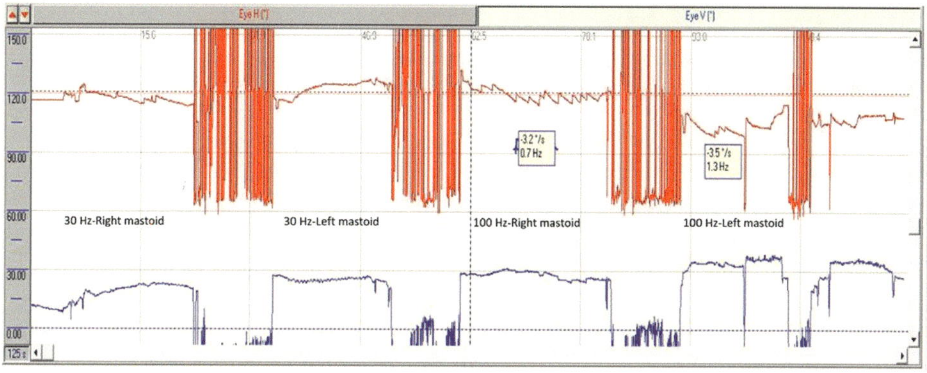

Figure 7.
The picture shows vibration-induced nystagmus (VIN) test results (SYNAPSYS VNG software by Inventis srl.) of a 45y female patient referred for her 5 years' history of vertigo attacks (about four attacks) associated with nausea and left-ear tinnitus. She had moderately severe SNHL in the left-ear. As you can see, the right-beating VIN provoked by performing 100 Hz vibration on both mastoids.

provokes more reliable VIN (average of 3.46°/s) compared with 30 Hz stimulus or stimulation of the unaffected ear [39]. Thus, this test can also help in MD diagnosis.

Additionally, the imbalance may present as unilateral weakness (UW) in the caloric test (**Figure 8**). Previous studies showed abnormal caloric results in 42–76% of MD patients [40].

Sometimes, the SN can also be seen (or even provoked) in Dix-Hallpike and/or positional tests. It is worthy to note that in some patients in attack phase, a direction-changing nystagmus can occur [41]. Consequently, we must be careful to distinguish these patients from others with benign paroxysmal positional vertigo (BPPV) or central type of positional vertigo.

The interesting thing to note is that the vestibular system also has a certain operating frequency. Some tests, such as caloric, cover a very low frequency range of the system (0.002–0.004 Hz), and some tests, such as vHIT, cover its high frequency range (5–7 Hz) [42]. Head-shaking test stimulates the vestibular system in the range

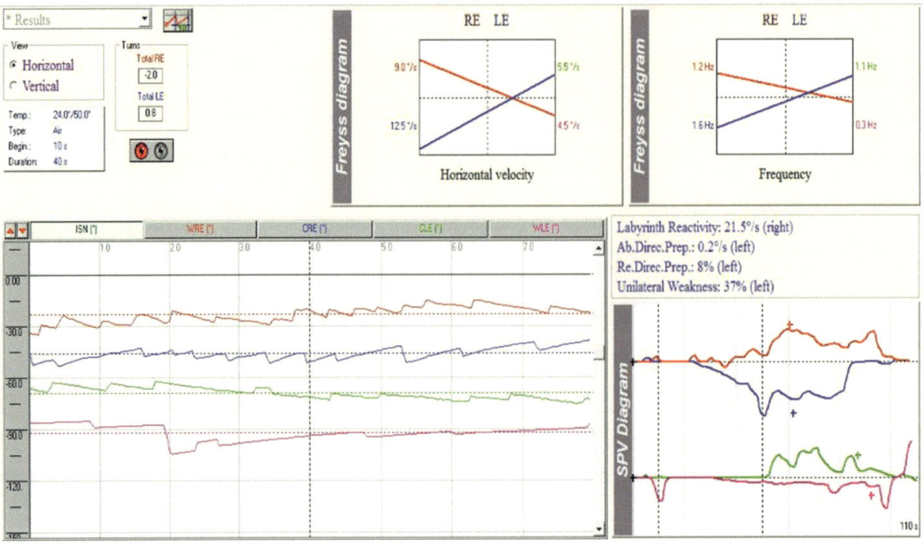

Figure 8.
The picture shows bi-thermal caloric test results (SYNAPSYS VNG software by Inventis srl.) of the patient presented in the **Figure 7***. Note the significant vestibular weakness in the ear (disordered side).*

of 1–2 Hz, and vibrational stimulus provokes the system in the range of 10–100 Hz [38]. Therefore, we can consider them as complementary tests that incite different population of vestibular hair cells and reinforce the diagnosis process.

3.2.2 Video head impulse test (vHIT)

During vHIT (or VHIT), a goggle with infrared camera placed on the patient's eyes or an infrared camera placed in front of the patient. The audiologist moves the patient's head quickly and unexpectedly in the horizontal and vertical planes to test horizontal and vertical semicircular canals (SCCs) and their neural pathways. In fact, six different movements are performed to test each of the six semicircular canals. The patient must keep his/her gaze on a front visual target. If the specific SCC works correctly, proper VOR will occur and the gaze will remain on the visual target. If the specific SCC does not work correctly, proper VOR will not occur and instead, corrective saccades will occur. VOR gain (eye velocity/head velocity) of >0.8 for horizontal SCCs and of >0.7 for vertical SCCs considered as normal response. Corrective saccades that occurred during head impulse (about 150 ms) or after head impulse called covert and overt saccades, respectively [40, 43, 44].

Several studies showed that vHIT results are usually normal in MD patients (**Figure 9**). On the other hand, a study by Lee et al. that analyzed HIT responses by magnetic search coil during MD attack showed that there is variation in the HIT results in terms of both the involved SCCs and the involved ear. Alongside, caloric results usually show some weakness on the affected side [45]. This dissociation may be due to how the vestibular system is stimulated during each test and cell types that involved by Meniere's disease [43, 45].

Anyway, as mentioned above, vHIT and caloric test are complementary for MD diagnosis.

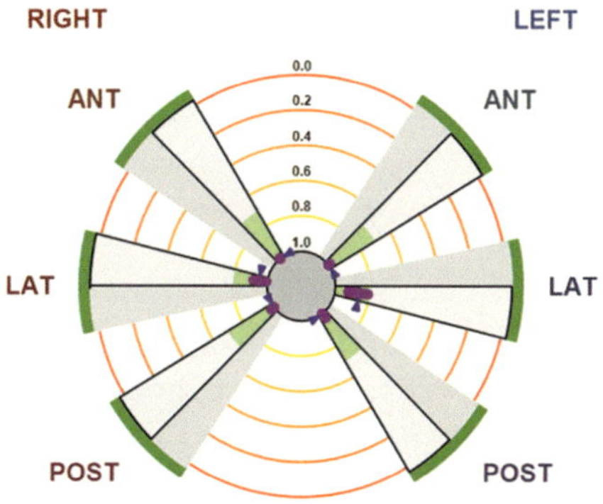

Impulses			VOR			Early saccades		
Canal		n	Mean gain	σ	Asymmetry	Ratio	Mean latency	Mean apparent gain
Ant.	R	10	1.11	0.03	2 %	0 %		
	L	10	1.07	0.04		0 %		
Lat.	R	12	0.95	0.02	5 %	0 %		
	L	15	0.86	0.03		0 %		
Post.	R	10	1.04	0.04	1 %	0 %		
	L	10	1.03	0.03		0 %		

Figure 9.
The picture shows video head impulse test (VHIT) results (SYNAPSYS VHIT software by Inventis srl.) of the patient presented in the **Figures 7** *and* **8**. *Note the normal VOR function in the plane of all six semicircular canals. However, sometimes a slight asymmetry can be seen between the results of the two sides, as presented in this case (VOR gain of 0.95 versus 0.86 for the right- and left-lateral SCCs, respectively).*

3.2.3 Subjective visual vertical/horizontal test (SVV/SVH)

During SVV/SVH, a luminous line projected on a screen and the patient must perceptually adjust it in vertical/horizontal plane. An error of more than ±2 degrees from the actual vertical or horizontal determined by the software is considered abnormal. This test can be performed in the upright or tilted head position; the latter is more sensitive to otolithic function [46].

In Meniere's disease, the results usually show tilt toward the affected ear, particularly in the acute phase. The results can be used to monitor the effects of surgery, treatment, or rehabilitation on the otolith function recovery [47, 48].

3.3 Vestibulo-spinal viewpoint

3.3.1 Posturography

Vestibulo-spinal function can be assessed by sensory organization test (SOT). SOT is a functional balance evaluation performed by posturography device. Posturography measures the postural sway and its parameters such as the direction, amplitude, velocity, and frequency [49]. The use of SOT may be helpful in the differential diagnosis of vestibular migraine from Meniere's disease [50].

SOT, caloric, and VHIT have a complementary role in evaluating VOR and VSR functions.

4. Conclusions

We have no specific test as "Meniere test," and its classification remains symptom-based. However, we often face with under-diagnosis or over-diagnosis. On the other hand, each audiological test has its own sensitivity and specificity in diagnosis of MD. Therefore, in addition to the symptoms, we must use a suitable and complementary set of hearing and vestibular tests to achieve the best diagnosis. We can look at MD from different perspectives that include: audiometry and aural symptoms, mechano-acoustic viewpoint, electro acoustic viewpoint, auditory electro-physiologic viewpoint, vestibular electro-physiologic viewpoint, vestibulo-ocular viewpoint, and vestibulo-spinal viewpoint.

Acknowledgements

I would like to thank my dear colleague, Dr. Farzam Jenabi (Audiologist), the esteemed director of the Department of Audiology (USWR), Professor Yones Lotfi (MD, ENT surgeon), and my respected colleagues at the comprehensive Clinic of Hearing and Balance at Rofeideh Rehabilitation Hospital.

I would like to express my sincere thanks to Inventis Company (Inventis srl.) for supporting the publication of this chapter.

Conflict of interest

Author Moslem Shaabani declares that he has received funding from a company Inventis srl. to cover the publication expenses for publishing this chapter. The Inventis srl. Did not fund the research presented in this work.

Author details

Moslem Shaabani
University of Social Welfare and Rehabilitation Sciences, Tehran, Iran

*Address all correspondence to: mo.shaabani@uswr.ac.ir

References

[1] Lee CS, Paparella MM, Margolis RH, Le C. Audiological profiles and Meniere's disease. Ear, Nose & Throat Journal. 1995;**74**(8):527-532

[2] Baloh RW. Prosper Meniere and his disease. Archives of Neurology. 2001;**58**(7):1151-1156

[3] Lopez-Escamez JA, Carey J, Chung WH, Goebel JA, Magnusson M, Mandalà M, et al. Diagnostic criteria for Menière's disease. Journal of Vestibular Research. 2015;**25**(1):1-7

[4] Basura GJ, Adams ME, Monfared A, Schwartz SR, Antonelli PJ, Burkard R, et al. Clinical practice guideline: Ménière's disease. Otolaryngology–Head and Neck Surgery. 2020;**162**(suppl. 2):S1-S55

[5] Zhang W, Hui L, Zhang B, Ren L, Zhu J, Wang F, et al. The correlation between endolymphatic hydrops and clinical features of Meniere disease. The Laryngoscope. 2021;**131**(1):E144-E150

[6] Savastano M, Guerrieri V, Marioni G. Evolution of audiometric pattern in Meniere's disease: Long-term survey of 380 cases evaluated according to the 1995 guidelines of the American Academy of Otolaryngology-Head and Neck Surgery. Journal of otolaryngology. 2006;**35**(1):26-29

[7] Committee on Hearing and Equilibrium. Committee on hearing and equilibrium guidelines for the diagnosis and evaluation of therapy in Meniere's disease. Otolaryngology–Head and Neck Surgery. 1995;**113**(3):181-185

[8] Mateijsen DJ, Van Hengel PW, Van Huffelen WM, Wit HP, Albers FW. Pure-tone and speech audiometry in patients with Menière's disease. Clinical Otolaryngology & Allied Sciences. 2001;**26**(5):379-387

[9] Frejo L, Soto-Varela A, Santos -Perez S, Aran I, Batuecas-Caletrio A, Perez-Guillen V, et al. Clinical subgroups in bilateral Meniere disease. Frontiers in Neurology. 2016;**7**:182

[10] Iacovou E, Vlastarakos PV, Ferekidis E, Nikolopoulos TP. Multi-frequency tympanometry: Clinical applications for the assessment of the middle ear status. Indian Journal of Otolaryngology and Head & Neck Surgery. 2013;**65**(3):283-287

[11] Meng X, Zhu K, Yue J, Han C. The role of wideband tympanometry in the diagnosis of Meniere's disease. Frontiers in Neurology. 2022;**13**:808921

[12] Sato E, Nakashima T, Lilly DJ, Fausti SA, Ueda H, Misawa H, et al. Tympanometric findings in patients with enlarged vestibular aqueducts. The Laryngoscope. 2002;**112**(9):1642-1646

[13] Lai D, Li W, Xian J, Liu S. Multifrequency tympanometry in adults with otitis media with effusion. European Archives of Oto-Rhino-Laryngology. 2008;**265**(9):1021-1025

[14] Miehe J, Mogensen S, Lyhne N, Skals R, Hougaard DD. Wideband tympanometry as a diagnostic tool for Menière's disease: A retrospective case-control study. European Archives of Oto-Rhino-Laryngology. 2022;**279**(4):1831-1841

[15] de Kleine E, Mateijsen DJ, Wit HP, Albers FW. Evoked otoacoustic emissions in patients with Ménière's disease. Otology & Neurotology. 2002;**23**(4):510-516

[16] Cunningham RF. Otoacoustic emissions: Beyond newborn hearing screening. Audiology Online. 2011:5

[17] Murdin L, Premachandra P, Davies R. Sensory dysmodulation in vestibular migraine: An otoacoustic emission suppression study. The Laryngoscope. 2010;**120**(8):1632-1636

[18] Albanese M, Di Girolamo S, Silvani L, Ciaschi E, Chiaramonte B, Conti M, et al. Distortion product Otoacoustic emissions and their suppression as predictors of peripheral auditory damage in migraine: A case-control study. Journal of Clinical Medicine. 2021;**10**(21):5007

[19] Chun RH, Pinto JM, Blankenhorn R, Dayal VS. Recovery of otoacoustic emission function in luetic endolymphatic hydrops: A possible measure of improvement in cochlear function. International Journal of Otolaryngology. 2009;**3**:2009

[20] van Tilburg MJ, Rauch SD. Electrophysiologic diagnosis of Meniere's disease. Current Otorhinolaryngology Reports. 2014;**2**(3):202-209

[21] Ferraro JA, Durrant JD. Electrocochleography in the evaluation of patients with Meniere's disease/ endolymphatic hydrops. Journal of the American Academy of Audiology. 2006;**17**(01):045-068

[22] Baba A, Takasaki K, Tanaka F, Tsukasaki N, Kumagami H, Takahashi H. Amplitude and area ratios of summating potential/action potential (SP/ AP) in Meniere's disease. Acta oto-laryngologica. 2009;**129**(1):25-29

[23] Hornibrook J. Tone burst electrocochleography for the diagnosis of clinically certain Meniere's disease. Frontiers in Neuroscience. 2017;**11**:301

[24] Park JH, Lee SY, Song JJ, Choi BY, Koo JW. Electrocochleographic findings in superior canal dehiscence syndrome. Hearing Research. 2015;**323**:61-67

[25] Martines F, Dispenza F, Montalbano C, Priola R, Torrente A, La Gumina R, et al. Comparison of electrocochleography and video head impulse test findings in vestibular migraine and Ménière disease: A preliminary study. The Journal of International Advanced Otology. 2020;**16**(2):183

[26] Kingma CM, Wit HP. Cochlear hydrops analysis masking procedure results in patients with unilateral Ménière's disease. Otology & Neurotology. 2010;**31**(6):1004-1008

[27] Wang HM, Tsai SM, Chien CY, Ho KY. Analysis of auditory and vestibular function in patients with unilateral Meniere's disease. Acta oto-laryngologica. 2012;**132**(12):1246-1251

[28] Young YH. Potential application of ocular and cervical vestibular-evoked myogenic potentials in Meniere's disease: A review. The Laryngoscope. 2013;**123**(2):484-491

[29] Shahnaz N, David EA. Normal values for cervical and ocular vestibular-evoked myogenic potentials using EMG scaling: Effect of body position and electrode montage. Acta Oto-Laryngologica. 2021;**141**(5):440-448

[30] Maxwell R, Jerin C, Gürkov R. Utilisation of multi-frequency VEMPs improves diagnostic accuracy for Meniere's disease. European Archives of Oto-Rhino-Laryngology. 2017;**274**(1):85-93

[31] Halmagyi GM. New clinical tests of unilateral vestibular dysfunction. The Journal of Laryngology & Otology. 2004;**118**(8):589-600

[32] Wang SJ, Weng WJ, Jaw FS, Young YH. Ocular and cervical vestibular-evoked myogenic potentials: A study to determine whether air-or bone-conducted stimuli are optimal. Ear and Hearing. 2010;**31**(2):283-288

[33] Angeli SI, Goncalves S. Cervical VEMP tuning changes by Meniere's disease stages. Laryngoscope Investigative Otolaryngology. 2019;**4**(5):543-549

[34] Curthoys IS, Vulovic V, Manzari L. Ocular vestibular-evoked myogenic potential (oVEMP) to test utricular function: Neural and oculomotor evidence. Acta Otorhinolaryngologica Italica. 2012;**32**(1):41

[35] Bery AK, Chang TP. Teaching video Neuroimages: Spontaneous nystagmus reversal in acute attack of ménière's disease. Neurology. 2020

[36] Kim MB, Huh SH, Ban JH. Diversity of head shaking nystagmus in peripheral vestibular disease. Otology & Neurotology. 2012;**33**(4):634-639

[37] Boniver R. Head-shaking nystagmus. B ENT. 2008;**3**:9-12

[38] Dumas G, Curthoys IS, Lion A, Perrin P, Schmerber S. The skull vibration-induced nystagmus test of vestibular function—A review. Frontiers in Neurology. 2017;**8**:41

[39] Dehkordi EM, Shaabani M, Kouhi A, Vahedi M. Vibration-induced nystagmus in patients with chronic unilateral Meniere's disease. Auditory and Vestibular Research. 2021;**30**(4):287-293

[40] Blödow A, Heinze M, Bloching MB, von Brevern M, Radtke A, Lempert T. Caloric stimulation and video-head impulse testing in Ménière's disease and vestibular migraine. Acta oto-laryngologica. 2014;**134**(12):1239-1244

[41] Noh H, Lee DH, Shin JE, Kim CH. Positional nystagmus after acute vertiginous attack in Meniere's disease. Audiology Research. 2021;**11**(1):55-62

[42] Weber KP, MacDougall HG, Halmagyi GM, Curthoys IS. Impulsive testing of semicircular-canal function using video-oculography. Annals of the New York Academy of Sciences. 2009;**1164**(1):486-491

[43] Limviriyakul S, Luangsawang C, Suvansit K, Prakairungthong S, Thongyai K, Atipas S. Video head impulse test and caloric test in definite Ménière's disease. European Archives of Oto-Rhino-Laryngology. 2020;**277**(3):679-686

[44] Kaci B, Nooristani M, Mijovic T, Maheu M. Usefulness of video head impulse test results in the identification of Meniere's disease. Frontiers in Neurology. 2020;**29**(11):581527

[45] Lee SU, Kim HJ, Koo JW, Kim JS. Comparison of caloric and head-impulse tests during the attacks of Meniere's disease. The Laryngoscope. 2017;**127**(3):702-708

[46] Winnick A, Sadeghpour S, Otero-Millan J, Chang TP, Kheradmand A. Errors of upright perception in patients with vestibular migraine. Frontiers in Neurology. 2018;**30**(9):892

[47] Toupet M, Van Nechel C, Grayeli AB. Influence of body laterality on recovery from subjective visual vertical tilt after vestibular neuritis. Audiology and Neurotology. 2014;**19**(4):248-255

[48] Shiozaki T, Wada Y, Ito T, Yamanaka T, Kitahara T. Changes in the results of the subjective visual vertical

test after endolymphatic sac drainage for intractable Meniere's disease. The Journal of International Advanced Otology. 2021;**17**(2):121-126

[49] Mohammadi M, Enayati Z, Shaabani M, Vahedi M. Stationary auditory white noise improves postural control in healthy adults: A novel study on head-shaking. Journal of Vestibular Research: Equilibrium & Orientation. 2022;**32**(2):99-112

[50] Hong HR, Shim DB, Kim TS, Shim BS, Ahn JH, Chung JW, et al. Results of caloric and sensory organization testing of dynamic posturography in migrainous vertigo: Comparison with Meniere's disease and vestibular neuritis. Acta Oto-Laryngologica. 2013;**133**(12):1236-1241

Chapter 7

Audio-Vestibular Side Effects of Drugs and Vaccines in Treatment of COVID-19

Magdalena B. Skarżyńska

Abstract

Due to the pandemic of COVID-19, a few new drugs and vaccines were officially approved by the EMA (European Medical Agency) and FDA (Food and Drug Administration) for prevention and treatment of SARS-CoV-2. The aim of this study is to analyze and highlight their potential audio-vestibular side effects as an ototoxic adverse reaction. The chapter was written by the review of the available literature in the scientific databases such as PubMed, ResearchGate, Scopus, and ScienceDirect, and in summaries of product characteristics as an official source of information. There were 39 publications and 15 summaries of product characteristics (as other sources of data), which were also used in this analysis. Adverse events could be permanent or disappear over time. Following treatment for COVID-19, the most frequent adverse audio-vestibular reactions reported in clinical trials and publications in the area of audiology and otorhinolaryngology were dizziness, blurry vision with dizziness, nasopharyngitis, dysgeusia, and tinnitus. As far as vaccines are concerned, dizziness as an ototoxic effect was uncommon and occurs only in hypersensitive people who experience anaphylactic shock. However, there is still a need to monitor ototoxic side effects because of potential interactions with other ototoxic drugs.

Keywords: ototoxicity, COVID-19 vaccine, audio-vestibular side effects, COVID-19 drugs, tinnitus

1. Introduction

The main aim of this chapter is to draw attention to the pharmacological treatments (medications and vaccines) for COVID-19 and the side effect. The number of patients who were treated and vaccinated against COVID-19 is very high. It is very important due to the fact that during clinical trials when the number of participants is limited, it is not always possible to detect every single adverse reaction of drug. Additionally, the participants in clinical trials are included after meeting the specific inclusion criteria. After approval of the drug, the treated population is more different (e.g., extensive or poor metabolizers). The potential audio-vestibular side effect as an ototoxic adverse effect was analyzed in relation to drugs that were currently approved by the EMA (European Medical Agency) and FDA (Food and Drug

IntechOpen

Administration) for the treatment of COVID-19. Some of the drugs and vaccines for the treatment of COVID-19 are new, and sometimes it is hard to predict every side effect. The number of patients in the 1, 2, and 3 phases of clinical trials is limited. As a result, some side effects may be observed during the IV phase (post-market surveillance). The detection risk and adverse events in this phase are possible due to the real-world usage of each drug. Adverse reactions are classified by the World Health Organization (WHO), and the probability of the occurrence of side effect is defined as follows: (1) very common ($\geq$ 1/10), (2) common ($\geq$ 1/100 to < 1/10), (3) uncommon ($\geq$ 1/1000 to < 1/100), (4) rare ($\geq$ 1/10000 to < 1/1000), (5) very rare (<1/10000), and the last, not known, which means that the frequency cannot be estimated from the available data.

The audio-vestibular side effects of drugs are classified as ototoxic side effects. Tinnitus, vertigo, and dizziness are examples of audio-vestibular side effects that should be considered during treatment for COVID-19. However, drugs and vaccines in the treatment of COVID-19 may cause the side effects in the area of the audio-vestibular area, the SARS-CoV-2 may itself manifest in the similar way. Similarly, COVID-19 disease may be linked to such audio-vestibular disorders as hearing loss, vertigo, dizziness, and/or tinnitus. There are a few hypotheses that are postulated. First is neuritis or cochleitis caused by the viral involvement of the vestibulocochlear nerve or inner ear. Second is vascular disorders, which may affect semicircular canals and cochlea by ischemia. The next purpose may be because of the production of the proinflammatory cytokines or microvascular injuries in the region of the peripheral and central nervous system that may be caused by the endothelial dysfunction. The last purpose may be connected with the accidental after cross-reaction of antibodies or T-cells damage to the inner ear [1]. Otorhinolaryngologists, neurologists, audiological specialists, and general practitioners should be aware of this. Tinnitus may manifest as sensorineural hearing loss (SNHL) or may be a consequence of central alterations caused by drugs. Vestibular side effects may manifest as loss of balance and dizziness, instability, unsteadiness, and difficulties in maintaining an upright posture [2, 3]. In many cases, it is difficult to find out if the source of the clinical symptoms is drug or the transition of the disease of COVID-19.

2. Material and methods

The analysis of the audio-vestibular adverse reactions of the treatment of COVID-19 was based on the identification of the relevant literature searching and the summaries of product characteristics of the drugs, which were officially approved by Food and Drug Administration (FDA) and European Medical Agency (EMA). From the analysis of adverse reactions of treatments and based on Evidence-Based Medicine (EBM), those drugs were eliminated from the analysis: chloroquine and hydroxychloroquine, favipiravir, lopinavir/ritonavir, amantadine, oseltamivir, azithromycin, and ivermectin. All of these drugs, even if at the beginning of the pandemic of COVID-19, were administered to patients and now are no longer recommended for treatment of COVID-19 due to a lack of clinical data, publications, and recommendation. The number and the type of drugs that are used at the same time in the treatment of COVID-19 depend on many different factors, such as: the severity of the disease, comorbidities, or other drugs that may interact with anti-COVID-19 drugs (e.g., PF-07321332/ritonavir). The terms of searching were as follows: SARS-CoV-2, COVID-19, audio-vestibular side effects, dizziness, ototoxicity, dexamethasone, anakinra, molnupiravir, tocilizumab, casirivimab and imdevimab, bamlanivimab and etesevimab, remdesivir, PF-07321332 and ritonavir, tixagevimab and cilgavimab, sotrovimab, and COVID-19 vaccines. The criteria of analyzed and inclusion were: (1) language (English), (2) type of studies (double-blinded, randomized), (3) the number of participants in the study. During the analysis of the adverse reactions, it is important to prove correlation between the presence of clinical symptoms with the exact drug or vaccine.

3. The results

To this moment, EMA has authorized 10 treatments against COVID-19, which were authorized: (1) tixagevimab and cilgavimab (2) casirivimab and imdevimab, (3) sotrovimab (4) regdanvimab, (5) tocilizumab, (6) PF-07321332 and ritonavir, (7) remdesivir, (8) anakinra, (9) molnupiravir, and (10) dexamethasone. FDA additionally approved bamlanivimab and etesevimab in the treatment of COVID-19. Most frequently reported adverse reactions following COVID-19 treatment in terms of the audio-vestibular disorders were dizziness, blurry vision with dizziness, nasopharyngitis, dysgeusia, and tinnitus [4]. All medications in the treatment of COVID-19 may be classified into one of the three groups: monoclonal antibodies, anti-viral drugs, and immunosuppressive agents.

Tixagevimab and cilgavimab are both recombinant human IgG1κ monoclonal antibodies, and the mechanism of action against SARS-CoV-2 is based on them binding to non-overlapping regions of receptor binding domain (RBD) of spike proteins. In total, 4220 subjects were enrolled in two clinical studies (PROVENT and STORM CHASER), where safety and efficiency were examined. In the area of audio-vestibular disorders, no side effects have so far been identified [5, 6]. Casirivimab and imdevimab are human immunoglobulin G1 (IgG1) antibodies that reduce endogenous immunoglobulin G levels by up to 79% [7, 8]. The effectiveness of the combination of these monoclonal antibodies was assessed on the results of a clinical trial of 799 adult participants with mild to moderate symptoms of COVID-19. For patients at high risk of developing severe disease, those treated with monoclonal antibodies had a reduced risk (3% versus 9%) of hospitalization or an emergency room visit within 28 days of starting treatment [9–12]. Sotrovimab is another monoclonal antibody (IgG1κ) with indication of treatment COVID-19 in adult and adolescents (above 12 years and weighing more than 40 kg), without requirement of supplemental oxygen but with the risk of progressing to severe phase of disease. The adverse reactions that were reported after administration of sotrovimab during phase II/III randomized, double-blind, and placebo-controlled clinical trial for treatment of COVID-19 in 1057 non-hospitalized, non-vaccinated adult patients (COMET-ICE clinical trial) include: hypersensitivity reactions (rash, bronchospasm), infusion-related reactions, and anaphylaxis, and dyspnea, but none of these can be classified as audio-vestibular disorders. The frequency of reported adverse reactions was classified as rare or uncommon. The adjusted relative risk reduction in hospitalization or death at 29 days of observation was 79% [13, 14].

Bamlanivimab is a recombinant, fully neutralizing human IgG monoclonal antibody. The mechanism of action based on the targeting RBD (receptor binding domain) of the spearhead protein. The information about the possible ototoxic effects of bamlanivimab is still limited, but dizziness may occur during and after of treatment with bamlanivimab according to the result of the clinical study BLAZE-1 (3.2% of patients reported an adverse event of dizziness) [15–18]. The combination of different monoclonal antibodies (tocilizumab and sarilumab – IL-6 receptor antagonists) in the clinical trials has been assessed in 803 adult patients: 353 patients in the "tocilizumab group," 48 patients in the sarilumab group and 402 patients, who were enrolled to the control group [19, 20]. Dizziness, as a type of ototoxicity side effect, is classified as common after treatment of tocilizumab [21, 22]. For sarilumab, according to the clinical trials and according to data, nasopharyngitis was reported as a common side effect [19, 23, 24].

Molnupiravir is an oral prodrug and treatment for COVID-19. Molnupiravir is a nucleotide analogue, which works by inhibiting the viral replication of the SARS-CoV-2 by causing viral mutagenesis [25]. The indication for molnupiravir is treatment of COVID-19 from mild to moderate in adult patients (COVID-19 positive patients) and those of them who are in the population of patients who are at the high risk of progressing the disease to severe phase. Molnupiravir is administered twice a day at the dose of 800 mg for 5 days. The effectiveness and safety were assessed in phase 3, double-blinded clinical trial (acronym MOVe-OUT) with 1411 non-hospitalized subjects, randomly divided into two subgroups: N = 710 (subjects that are treated with molnupiravir and N = 701 subjects as a control group (placebo group). During clinical trials, serious adverse reactions occurred in 7% in the first subgroup and in 10% of those patients from the placebo group. In the area of audio-vestibular disorders, dizziness was mostly reported and occurs in 1% of patients from both groups [25, 26]. The second oral anti-COVID-19 drug is the combination of co-packaged tablets with two active substances ritonavir and PF-07321332. PF-07321332 is a SARS-CoV-2 main protease (Mpro) inhibitor, and ritonavir is an HIV-1 protease inhibitor and CYP3A inhibitor [27]. The efficacy and safety of this drug were assessed in the randomized and placebo-controlled, phase 2/3 of the clinical trial (C4671005 EPIC-HR) with 2224 adult patients who suffer form COVID-19. Enrolled patients were then divided into two subgroups: the first one with 1109 patients and the second one with 1115 subjects. In total, 6% of all patients reported dysgeusia, and the most common side reactions were: hypertension, myalgia, and diarrhea [27].

Anakinra has been authorized for treatment of many diseases such as rheumatoid arthritis for adult patients, autoinflammatory periodic fever syndromes, and for treatment of *Cryopyrin-Associated Periodic Syndromes*. The mechanism of action of anakinra is based on neutralization of the biologic activity of interleukins (IL-1α and IL-1β) by inhibiting the binding to the receptor IL-1RI. The efficacy and safety of anakinra in the treatment of COVID-19 were assessed during randomized, placebo-controlled clinical trial with the acronym SAVE-MORE. In total, 405 patients were enrolled to this study. Side effects in the area of the otorhinolaryngology and audio-vestibular disorders were not [28, 29].

Dexamethasone has an anti-inflammatory effect and is therefore mainly used as an adjunct in the treatment of viral pneumonia. Due to its higher potency, it is suspected that this drug might prove effective in treating patients with SARS-CoV-2 [30–32]. Dexamethasone in the treatment of COVID-19 is responsible downgrading IDO1 (indoleamine 2,3-dioxygenase) and AhR (aryl hydrocarbon receptors) genes and as a result, reducing inflammation. After entering the human body, SARS-CoV-2 activates receptor AhR (aryl hydrocarbon receptors) after entering their target cells through a mechanism independent of IDO1. SAAS (systemic AhR activation syndrome) is the result of the upregulation of the series effectors that are depended on the AhR [30, 33, 34]. The strong recommendation for administration of dexamethasone in severe-ill patients is to prevent or reduce a systemic inflammatory response, which may lead to the multiorgan dysfunction and damage of the lung [35]. The European Medical Agency (EMA) approved dexamethasone for the treatment of

COVID-19 patients undergoing mechanical or aerobic ventilation [36]. Side effects in the area of otorhinolaryngology may cause blurry vision with dizziness [30, 35].

Remdesivir, which is an adenosine nucleotide prodrug, was one of the first drugs approved for the treatment of COVID-19. It is metabolized in the human organism into the remdesivir triphosphate and impacts on the replication of the viral RNA. The safety and efficacy were evaluated during NIAID ACTT-1 Study with 1063 participants. None of the audio-vestibular adverse reactions were reported [37].

3.1 COVID-19 vaccines

Until then, there are five vaccines approved by European Medical Agency: (1) Comirnaty (marketing authorization holder: BioNTech and Pfizer), (2) Nuvaxovid (marketing authorization holder: Novavax), (3) Spikevax (marketing authorization holder: Moderna), (4) Vaxzevria (marketing authorization holder: AstraZeneca), and (5) Jcovden (marketing authorization holder: Janssen). According to the data presented by EMA in safety report of COVID-19 vaccines, 870 million doses of vaccines have been given to citizens in the area of European Union (UE) and European Economic Area (EEA), and there is no information about the new audio-vestibular adverse reactions. The vast majority of all side effects are mild and short-lived [38]. Clinical trials show that systemic and local reactions may occur as a result of vaccination. According to the clinical data and what patients most frequently report are pain at the injection site and less frequently redness or swelling at the site, headache and fatigue, and fever. After official authorization of COVID-19 vaccines by European Medical Agency (EMA) and Food and Drug Administration (FDA), the continuation of monitoring and analysis of further side effects is obligation of pharmaceutical companies and safety authorities. Some of the drugs and vaccines for the treatment of COVID-19 are new, and sometimes it is hard to predict every side effect. The number of patients in the 1, 2, and 3 phases of clinical trials is limited. As a result, some side effects may be observed during the IV phase (post-market surveillance). The detection risk and adverse events in this phase are possible due to the real-world usage of each drug. Some authors highlight that there may be relationship between occurrence of tinnitus and SSNHL (Sudden Sensorineural Hearing Loss) after vaccination, but it needs further clinical studies and observation as the relationship has been described as indirect [39–41].

According to the summary of product characteristics, Comirnaty in one dose contains 30 μg of COVID-19 mRNA embedded in lipid nanoparticles. The efficacy and safety ratio of this vaccine was evaluated in participants enrolled in two clinical studies that included 21,744 participants who had received at least one dose of the vaccine. The most frequent side effects in participants that were reported are: (1) pain at the injection site (>80%), (2) fatigue (>60%), (3) headache (> 50%), (4) myalgia and chills (>30%), (5) arthralgia (>20 %), (6) pyrexia, and (7) swelling at the injection site (>10 %). The side effects were classified as mild to moderate and usually resolved within a few days after vaccination. Dizziness as an audio-vestibular side effect occurred only in hypersensitive people as part of anaphylactic shock, and its frequency is unknown (it cannot be estimated from available data) [42].

Moderna COVID-19 vaccine in one dose contains 100 μg of COVID-19 messenger RNA embedded in SM-102 lipid nanoparticles. The effectiveness and safety profile was evaluated in a randomized, placebo-controlled phase 3 clinical trial in 30,351 participants who received at least one dose of the vaccine. The most frequent reported adverse reactions in participants were similar as in all other vaccines: (1) pain at the injection site (92%), (2) fatigue (70%), (3) headache (64.7%), (3) myalgia (61.5%), (4) arthralgia (46.4%), (5) chills (45.4%), (6) nausea/vomiting (23%), (7) axillary swelling/tenderness (19.8%), (8) fever (15.5%), (9) swelling at the injection site (14.7%), and (10) redness (10%). The side effects were defined between mild to moderate and not long-lasting (usually side effects resolved in the period within a few days after injection). Dizziness as an ototoxic effect may occurred only in hypersensitive people as part of anaphylactic shock, and its frequency is unknown (cannot be estimated from the available data) [43].

One dose of vaccine consists of 0.5 mL (brand name: Vaxzevria. The efficacy and safety were assessed in four clinical trials with number of participants: 23,745. The most frequently reported adverse reactions were: (1) injection site tenderness (>60%); (2) injection site pain, (3) headache, (4) fatigue (>50%); (5) myalgia, (6) malaise (>40%); (7) pyrexia, (8) chills (>30%), (9) arthralgia, and (10) nausea (>20%). In the area of otorhinolaryngology, dizziness as an ototoxic side effect may occur only in people who are hypersensitive for the ingredients of vaccine as a part of anaphylactic shock. The frequency of the reaction is unknown [44–48].

Janssen vaccine is an adenovirus vaccine against COVID-19 disease, and one dose (0.5 mL) contains adenovirus type 26 encoding the SARS-CoV-2 spike glycoprotein* (Ad26.COV2-S, not less than 8.92 log10 infectious units). The safety of Janssen COVID-19 vaccine has been evaluated in an ongoing Phase 3 study (COV3001) in which a total of 21,895 adults aged 18 years and older received a single-dose vaccination. The most common systemic adverse reactions were: (1) headache (38.9%), (2) fatigue (38.2%), (3) myalgia (33.2%), and (4) nausea (14.2%). Pyrexia (body temperature $\geq$ 38.0°C) was observed in 9% of participants. The most important side effects in the audiology and otorhinolaryngology field reported in the clinical trials were dizziness (of uncommon frequency) and tinnitus (rare).

Nuvaxovid is a recombinant, adjuvanted vaccine against COVID-19, and one dose (0.5 mL) contains 5 μg of the SARS-CoV-2 spike protein and is adjuvanted with Matrix-M. The safety profile was evaluated from five clinical trials involving 49,950 adult participants. The adverse reactions were mild to moderate and included (1) site tenderness (75%), (2) injection site pain (62%), (3) fatigue (53%), (4) myalgia (51%), (5) headache (50%), (6) malaise (41%), (7) arthralgia (24%), (8) nausea, and (9) vomiting (15%). The duration of adverse reactions was a few days. No adverse reactions important from an otorhinolaryngological or audiological point of view were reported. Dizziness as an ototoxic effect occurred only in hypersensitive people as part of anaphylactic shock and as an adverse reaction with uncommon frequency [49].

4. Discussion and conclusion

At the beginning of pandemic of COVID-19 and due to the lack of specific treatment ototoxicity as a side effect was reported after treatment included chloroquine and hydroxychloroquine. By analyzing new, COVID-19 therapies, including those already approved by the regulatory authorities (EMA and FDA), we will be able to gain knowledge about new disease treatment protocols and their possible side effects, including those related to the hearing organ. The earlier we can implement monitoring measures the better. Patients with renal impairment, children under 3 years of age, people over 65 years of age, pregnant women, and patients who have been treated with ototoxic drugs or who will be administered an ototoxic drug for more than 14 days are at higher risk of presence of side effects [41, 50, 51]. Tinnitus, dizziness, vertigo are the most frequently reported side effects in the area of the audio-vestibular disorders during the treatment of COVID-19. This is important not only for specialist such as otorhinolaryngologists, audiologists, but also for neurologists and general practitioners. As far as tinnitus is concerned, this disorder may manifest as sensorineural hearing loss (SNHL). Loss of balance, dizziness, instability, difficulties in maintaining an upright posture, and unsteadiness are classified as vestibular side effects.

In 2021, the FDA and EMA approved monoclonal antibodies and oral drugs for treatment of COVID-19. The SARS-CoV-2 itself may cause similar audio-vestibular disorders. Many of the drugs approved by the EMA and FDA are new, and as a result not every side effect is known. Dizziness, blurry vision with dizziness, and tinnitus are the most frequently reported adverse reactions during and after treatment of the COVID-19. Additionally, nasopharyngitis and dysgeusia have been reported. While vaccines are concerned, dizziness as an ototoxic effect may occur only in hypersensitive people as a result of anaphylactic shock (a rare adverse reaction). The ototoxicity (hearing loss) of the drugs described in this chapter does not have such severe symptoms as some drugs used in the treatment of COVID-19 in 2020 (in particular, hydroxychloroquine). The continuous monitoring of possible ototoxic side effects may arise from interactions with other ototoxic drugs. Finally, the SARS-CoV-2 itself may cause similar audio-vestibular disorders as the drugs for treatment of COVID-19.

Author details

Magdalena B. Skarżyńska[1,2,3]

1 Hospital Pharmacy, Poland

2 Institute of Sensory Organs, Kajetany, Poland

3 Center of Hearing and Speech, Kajetany, Poland

*Address all correspondence to: m.skarzynska@csim.pl

References

[1] Di Mauro P, La Mantia I, Cocuzza S, Sciancalepore PI, Rasà D, Maniaci A, et al. Acute Vertigo after COVID-19 vaccination: Case series and literature review. Frontiers in Medicine. 2022;**8**;2766-2771

[2] Altissimi G, Colizza A, Cianfrone G, Vincentiis MD, Greco A, Taurone S, et al. Drugs Inducing Hearing Loss, Tinnitus, Dizziness and Vertigo: An Updated Guide. European Review for Medical and Pharmacological Sciences. 2020;**24**:7946-7952

[3] Seligmann H, Podoshin L, Ben-David J, Fradis M, Goldsher M. Drug-induced tinnitus and other hearing disorders. Drug Safety. 1996;**14**:198-212. DOI: 10.2165/00002018-199614030-00006

[4] Skarzynska MB, Matusiak M, Skarzynski PH. Adverse Audio-vestibular effects of drugs and vaccines used in the treatment and prevention of COVID-19: A review. Audiology Research. 2022;**12**:224-248. DOI: 10.3390/audiolres12030025

[5] AstraZeneca. Tixagevimab Co-Packaged with Cilgavimab–Fact Sheet For Healthcare Providers: Emergency Use Authorization For Evusheld. 2021. Available online: https://www.fda.gov/media/154701/download

[6] Levin MJ, Ustianowski A, De Wit S, Launay O, Avila M, Seegobin S, et al. LB5. PROVENT: Phase 3 Study of Efficacy and Safety of AZD7442 (Tixagevimab/Cilgavimab) for Pre-Exposure Prophylaxis of COVID-19 in Adults. Open Forum Infectious Diseases. 2021;**8**:S810. DOI: 10.1093/ofid/ofab466.1646

[7] Casirivimab. Drugs and Lactation Database (LactMed). Bethesda (MD): National Library of Medicine (US); 2006

[8] Imdevimab. In Drugs and Lactation Database (LactMed). Bethesda (MD): National Library of Medicine (US); 2006

[9] Casirivimab and Imdevimab. Available online: https://www.regeneron.com/medicines/casirivimab-imdevimab. [Accessed January 19, 2022]

[10] REGEN-COV® (Casirivimab and Imdevimab) Official HCP Site. Available online: https://www.regencov.com/hcp. [Accessed January 19, 2022]

[11] Commissioner, O. of the Coronavirus (COVID-19) Update: Daily Roundup. 2020 Available online: https://www.fda.gov/news-events/press-announcements/coronavirus-covid-19-update-daily-roundup-march-24-2020. [Accessed January 19, 2022]

[12] Weinreich DM, Sivapalasingam S, Norton T, Ali S, Gao H, Bhore R, et al. REGEN-COV antibody combination and outcomes in outpatients with Covid-19. The New England Journal of Medicine. 2021;**385**:e81. DOI: 10.1056/NEJMoa2108163

[13] GlaxoSmithKline Manufacturing S.p.A. Sotrovimab–Summary of Product Characteristics. 2021. Available online: https://www.ema.europa.eu/en/documents/product-information/xevudy-epar-product-information_en.pdf

[14] Gupta A, Gonzalez-Rojas Y, Juarez E, Crespo Casal M, Moya J, Falci DR, et al. Early treatment for Covid-19 with SARS-CoV-2 neutralizing antibody Sotrovimab. New England Journal of Medicine.

2021;**385**:1941-1950. DOI: 10.1056/NEJMoa2107934

[15] An EUA for Bamlanivimab. A Monoclonal Antibody for COVID-19. JAMA. 2021;**325**:880-881. DOI: 10.1001/jama.2020.24415

[16] FDA Issues EUA for Bamlanivimab to Treat COVID-19. Available online: http://www.pharmacist.com/Pharmacy-News/fda-issues-eua-for-bamlanivimab-to-treat-covid-19. [Accessed January 9, 2022]

[17] Bamlanivimab and Etesevimab Emergency Use Authorization (EUA) for COVID-19. Available online: https://www.covid19.lilly.com/bam-ete/hcp. [Accessed January 19, 2022]

[18] Dougan M, Nirula A, Azizad M, Mocherla B, Gottlieb RL, Chen P, et al. Bamlanivimab plus Etesevimab in Mild or Moderate Covid-19. New England Journal of Medicine. 2021;**385**:1382-1392. DOI: 10.1056/NEJMoa2102685

[19] Gordon AC, Mouncey PR, Al-Beidh F, Rowan KM, Nichol AD, Arabi YM, et al. Interleukin-6 receptor antagonists in critically ill patients with Covid-19. The New England Journal of Medicine. 2021:1491-1502

[20] COVID Research: A Year of Scientific Milestones. Nature. 2021. DOI: 10.1038/d41586-020-00502-w. Available online: https://www.nature.com/articles/d41586-020-00502-w

[21] Anonymous RoActemra. Available online: https://www.ema.europa.eu/en/medicines/human/EPAR/roactemra

[22] Roche Registration GmbH Roactemra - Summary of Product Characteristics 2022

[23] Kevzara 150 Mg Solution for Injection in Pre-Filled Syringe - Summary of Product Characteristics (SmPC) - (Emc). Available online: https://www.medicines.org.uk/emc/product/762/smpc#gref. [Accessed January 19, 2022]

[24] Stone JH, Frigault MJ, Serling-Boyd NJ, Fernandes AD, Harvey L, Foulkes AS, et al. Efficacy of tocilizumab in patients hospitalized with Covid-19. New England Journal of Medicine. 2020;**383**:2333-2344. DOI: 10.1056/NEJMoa2028836

[25] Merck & Co., Inc. Molnupiravir—Fact Sheet for Healthcare Providers: Emergency Use Authorization; New York, NY, USA: Merck & Co., Inc.; 2022

[26] Covid-19: Molnupiravir Reduces Risk of Hospital Admission or Death by 50% in Patients at Risk, MSD Reports | The BMJ. Available online: https://www.bmj.com/content/375/bmj.n2422. [Accessed: February 17, 2022]

[27] Pfizer Labs Paxlovid: Fact Sheet For Healthcare Providers: Emergency Use Authorization. 2022. Available online: https://www.fda.gov/media/155050/download

[28] Boehringer Ingelheim RCV GmbH & Co KG. Pfizer Health AB Kineret–Summary of Product Characteristics. Wien, Austria: Boehringer Ingelheim RCV GmbH & Co KG; 2021

[29] Kyriazopoulou E, Poulakou G, Milionis H, Metallidis S, Adamis G, Tsiakos K, et al. Early treatment of COVID-19 with Anakinra guided by soluble urokinase plasminogen receptor plasma levels: A double-blind, randomized controlled phase 3 Trial. Nature Medicine. 2021;**2021**:27, 1752. DOI: 10.1038/s41591-021-01499-z

[30] Ahmed MH, Hassan A. Dexamethasone for the treatment of Coronavirus Disease (COVID-19):

A review. SN comprehensive clinical medicine. 2020:1-10. DOI: 10.1007/s42399-020-00610-8

[31] Becker DE. Basic and clinical pharmacology of glucocorticosteroids. Anesthesia Progress. 2013;**60**:25-31

[32] Zoorob RJ, Cender D. A different look at corticosteroids. American Family Physician. 1998;**58**:443-450

[33] Li F, Li W, Farzan M, Harrison SC. Structure of SARS coronavirus spike receptor-binding domain complexed with receptor. Science. 2005;**309**:1864-1868

[34] Turski WA, Wnorowski A, Turski GN, Turski CA, Turski L. AhR and IDO1 in pathogenesis of Covid-19 and the "Systemic AhR Activation Syndrome:" A Translational Review and Therapeutic Perspectives. Restorative Neurology and Neuroscience. 2020;**38**:343-354. DOI: 10.3233/RNN-201042

[35] RECOVERY Collaborative Group, Horby P, Lim WS, Emberson JR, Mafham M, Bell JL, et al. Dexamethasone in hospitalized patients with Covid-19. The New England Journal of Medicine. 2021;**384**:693-704. DOI: 10.1056/NEJMoa2021436

[36] Czarska-Thorley D. Ema endorses Use of Dexamethasone in COVID-19 Patients on Oxygen or Mechanical Ventilation. Available online: https://www.ema.europa.eu/en/news/ema-endorses-use-dexamethasone-covid-19-patients-oxygen-mechanical-ventilation. [Accessed: January 19, 2022]

[37] Gilead Sciences Ireland UC Remdesivir – Summary of Product Characteristics. 2022. Available online: https://www.ema.europa.eu/en/medicines/human/EPAR/veklury

[38] EMA Safety of COVID-19 Vaccines Available online: https://www.ema.europa.eu/en/human-regulatory/overview/public-health-threats/coronavirus-disease-covid-19/treatments-vaccines/vaccines-covid-19/safety-covid-19-vaccines. [Accessed May 21, 2022]

[39] Thrane JF, Britze A, Fjaeldstad AW. Incidence and Duration of Self-Reported Hearing Loss and Tinnitus in a Cohort of COVID-19 Patients with Sudden Chemosensory Loss: A STROBE Observational Study – ScienceDirect. Available online: https://www.sciencedirect.com/science/article/pii/S1879729621002246. [Accessed February 20, 2022]

[40] Jeong J, Choi HS. Sudden sensorineural hearing loss after COVID-19 vaccination. International Journal of Infectious Diseases. 2021;**113**:341-343. DOI: 10.1016/j.ijid.2021.10.025

[41] Ciorba A, Corazzi V, Skarżyński PH, Skarżyńska MB, Bianchini C, Pelucchi S, et al. Don't forget ototoxicity during the SARS-CoV-2 (Covid-19) pandemic! International Journal of Immunopathology and Pharmacology. 2020;**34**:205. DOI: 10.1177/2058738420941754

[42] COMIRNATY®▼ | Pfizer UK. Available online: https://www.pfizer.co.uk/products/prescription-medicines/comirnaty. [Accessed January 19, 2022]

[43] Summary of Product Characteristics for Spikevax. Available online: https://www.gov.uk/government/publications/regulatory-approval-of-covid-19-vaccine-moderna/information-for-healthcare-professionals-on-covid-19-vaccine-moderna. [Accessed January 19, 2022]

[44] AstraZeneca's COVID-19 Vaccine Authorised for Emergency Supply

in the UK. Available online: https://www.astrazeneca.com/media-centre/press-releases/2020/astrazenecas-covid-19-vaccine-authorised-in-uk.html. [Accessed January 19, 2022]

[45] CDC Ensuring the Safety of COVID-19 Vaccines in the United States. Available online: https://www.cdc.gov/coronavirus/2019-ncov/vaccines/safety.html. [Accessed January 9, 2022]

[46] Tseng P-T, Chen T-Y, Sun Y-S, Chen Y-W, Chen J-J. The reversible tinnitus and cochleopathy followed first-dose astrazeneca COVID-19 vaccination. QJM. 2021;**114**:663-664. DOI: 10.1093/qjmed/hcab210

[47] Regulatory Approval of Vaxzevria (Previously COVID-19 Vaccine AstraZeneca) Available online: https://www.gov.uk/government/publications/regulatory-approval-of-covid-19-vaccine-astrazeneca. [Accessed January 19, 2022]

[48] Falsey AR, Sobieszczyk ME, Hirsch I, Sproule S, Robb ML, Corey L, et al. Phase 3 safety and efficacy of AZD1222 (ChAdOx1 NCoV-19) Covid-19 vaccine. New England Journal of Medicine. 2021;**385**:2348-2360. DOI: 10.1056/NEJMoa2105290

[49] Novavax CZ a.s. Nuvaxovid-Summary of Product Characteristics. 2022. Available online: https://www.ema.europa.eu/en/documents/product-information/nuvaxovid-epar-product-information_en.pdf?_x_tr_sl=en&_x_tr_tl=fi&_x_tr_hl=fi&_x_tr_pto=sc

[50] Rybak LP. Ototoxicity of loop diuretics. Otolaryngologic Clinics of North America. 1993;**26**:829-844

[51] Savitz DA, Styka AN, editors. National Academies of Sciences, Engineering, and Medicine Assessment of Long-Term Health Effects of Antimalarial Drugs When Used for Prophylaxis. Washington, DC: The National Academies Press; 2020